Total Quality Service in Healthcare

Total Quality Service in Healthcare

An Empirical Investigation

Usha Manjunath

Rawat Publications

Jaipur • New Delhi • Bangalore • Hyderabad • Guwahati

ISBN 978-81-316-0469-4

The publication of this book was financially supported by the ICSSR. The responsibility for the facts stated, opinions expressed, or conclusions reached, is entirely that of the author and that the ICSSR accepts no responsibility for them.

ICSSR Consultant: Professor V. Venkaiah, Dr B.R. Ambedkar Open University, Hyderabad (A.P.)

Published by
Prem Rawat for **Rawat Publications**
Satyam Apts, Sector 3, Jawahar Nagar, Jaipur 302 004 (India)
Phone: 0141 265 1748 / 7006 Fax: 0141 265 1748
E-mail: info@rawatbooks.com
Website: www.rawatbooks.com

New Delhi Office
4858/24, Ansari Road, Daryaganj, New Delhi 110 002
Phone: 011 2326 3290

Also at *Bangalore, Hyderabad* and *Guwahati*

Typeset by Rawat Computers, Jaipur
Printed at Nice Printing Press, New Delhi

In memory of my

Mother and Father

the yin and yang of my existence

Contents

	Acknowledgements	ix
	Preface	xiii
1	Introduction to Quality Management in Healthcare Organizations	1
2	Core Issues in Healthcare Quality	17
3	Quality Assurance in Healthcare	31
4	Total Quality Management in Healthcare	49
5	Quality Management of Healthcare Services in India	71
6	Research on Quality Dimensions for TQS Implementation	91
7	Validating Quality Constructs: Observations from Studies in Indian Hospitals	117
8	Empirical Investigation of TQS	142

9 Integrative Framework for Total Quality Service Management in Hospitals 166

10 Conclusions and Future Research Directions 184

Appendices 197

References 247

Index 269

Acknowledgements

I sincerely express my gratitude to Prof. L.K. Maheshwari, Former Vice Chancellor, BITS, Pilani, for having permitted to pursue my research work at BITS. I take this opportunity to thank Prof. G. Raghurama, Director, BITS, Pilani, for providing me the necessary facilities required for carrying out the research work and all his support and encouragement. My special thanks to Dr K.S. Srinivasa Rao, Director, Institute of Health Management Research, Bangalore, for providing the necessary Institutional support for publishing the thesis work in this book form.

I express my heartfelt gratitude to my revered guide Prof. Anil K. Bhat, Management Studies Group, BITS, Pilani, for his unmitigated support and more importantly, for being my research supervisor. His meticulous reviews, in-depth inquiry and advice on the work have added immense value to the thesis.

My special thanks to Dr R.P. Pareek, Medical Superintendent, Medical Centre, BITS, Pilani, for his valuable suggestions and guidance during my studies in Hospital and Health System Management.

I would like to express my sincere thanks to Prof. B.A. Metri, Associate Professor and Chairperson PG Programme, MDI, Gurgaon, for all his expert guidance and suggestions at the various stages of my research work. I have great pleasure in recording my gratitude to Prof. N.V.M. Rao, Economics and Finance Group, Dean, Hardware Division, BITS, Pilani, for all his help during data collection, analysis and writing of the thesis work.

I express my deep sense of gratitude to all the senior managers of 40 major hospitals in India who participated in various stages of the study. Special thanks to the following doctors and managers who helped me obtain necessary contacts/permissions for the study and provided expert inputs and participated in lengthy interviews:

- Dr G. Bakthavalsalam, Chairman, Mr Christopher Francis, Human Resources Development Manager and Dr T. Ramachandran, Senior Consultant K.G. Hospital, Coimbatore
- Dr Father Sabastian, Associate Director and Dr A. Mohan, Prof. and HOD, Urology, St. John's Medical College Hospital, Bangalore
- Dr Satish Amarnath, Microbiologist and QMR, and Dr K.G. Shetty, Director, Clinical Services, Manipal Hospital, Bangalore
- Dr Madan Gaekwad, Vice President, Sagar Apollo Hospital, Bangalore
- Dr Murali Mohan, General Manager, Hospital Operations, SVIMS, Tirupati
- Dr Capt. K. Narasimha, Company Medical Officer, Company Medical Officer Harita TVS Technologies Limited
- Dr S. Biswas, Apollo Gleneagles Hospital, Kolkata
- Dr Subramanya, Ex. Founder Chairman, Bangalore Hospital, Bangalore
- Dr Raghavendra Chikkatur, Cardiothoracic Surgeon, Sri Jayadeva Institute of Cardiovascular Sciences & Research, Bangalore
- Dr Kishore Murthy, Former CEO, Bhagwan Mahavir Jain Hospital, Bangalore
- Dr Nitish Shetty, Group CEO, Narayana Dental Chain and Mr Kishore Reddy, Head, Telemedicine, Narayana Hrudayalaya, Bangalore
- Dr Jayashree Bhat, Associate Professor, KMC Hospital, Mangalore

- Dr Murali Chakravarti, Anaesthesiologist, Wockhardt Hospital Pvt. Ltd., Bangalore
- Dr H.V. Srinivas, Ophthalmologist, Aditya Eye Clinic, Bangalore
- Mr Uday Naik, Administrator, Bangalore Institute of Oncology, Bangalore
- Mr Venkat Panidhar, Chief Hospital Administrator, NRI Medical College Hospital, Vijayawada

My friends Dr Sangeeta Sharma, Dr B. Geetha, Dr Jayashree Bhat, Dr Ravi Kumar, Dr Gajendra Chauhan, Ms. Kathyayini Venkatesh and Dr Monica Sharma were there to support through tough times and encouraged me constantly, always.

During these four years of long hours of work and ups and downs, my family and friends stood by me. My husband Manjunath and daughter Sindhu need special mention for putting up with my crazy working hours and preoccupations.

I express my profound gratitude to the Indian Council of Social Science Research for providing the financial assistance for publishing the research thesis in the book form. I am highly indebted to Rawat Publications, Jaipur and particularly Mr Pranit Rawat of Rawat Publications for their fine editorial help in guiding and producing this book.

Preface

The healthcare industry, a critical development sector, across the world presents a very dynamic and an uncertain environment. The healthcare system in India is fast evolving and expanding. The sector presents a mixed picture in terms of quality and reach. A vast majority of private high-tech care is concentrated in urban centres, and the rural areas are underserviced. Though there are centres of excellence in healthcare delivery, many areas of the nation suffers from poor health infrastructure. Quality of services in the highly fragmented sector is variable and the regulatory mechanisms are inadequate.

The central theme of all healthcare systems is 'quality' and it needs to be managed effectively for their survival and performance excellence in today's business environment. Operationalization of the concepts of quality at the organizational level has led to several innovations in quality management, from the traditional quality assurance to implementation of the philosophy of Total Quality Management (TQM). For effective implementation of TQM in an organization, it is important to identify critical quality management strategies. The literature on quality management implies that when decision-makers in an organization focus on better management of the critical factors, improvements in the quality of the products or services will occur. And ultimately, such efforts will result in improved organizational performance in terms of financial indicators, customer loyalty and satisfaction. Further, the researchers can use such operational measures to build theories and models for quality management.

Research on critical success factors for TQM implementation in non-healthcare context is quite well established. In fact, the application of TQM and Continuous Quality Improvements has provided a boost to the manufacturing sector at large. Implementation and research in total quality in healthcare has been a major focus in many of the developed nations. In the Indian context, professional management of hospitals has increasingly gained importance since 1990s, but research on Total Quality Service (TQS) Management is very limited. The present study is an attempt towards further refinement of TQS constructs for the hospital sector from a managerial perspective.

This research work closely examines merits and demerits of many quality assurance mechanisms in healthcare and makes a strong case for the implementation of TQM in healthcare. The empirical investigation of critical success factors (or quality constructs) of total quality in hospitals in India and the development of a conceptual Integrative Total Quality Service Management Framework are detailed in this book.

We hope that this book will reach a wider audience and provide decision-makers, academicians and researchers many concepts and tools in 'healthcare quality' and contribute significantly to healthcare quality management literature in the Indian context.

Dr Usha Manjunath
Associate Professor and Chairperson-Academics
Institute of Health Management Research
Bangalore

1

Introduction to Quality Management in Healthcare Organizations

In the last two decades, the service sector is emerging as one of the biggest and fastest growing sectors in world economy including India. Societies are increasingly looking at 'quality of life' enhancements through various services such as better government services, infrastructure, education, healthcare, public utility and so on. India has seen a major growth since 1991, the year known for opening up of economy and liberalization. In the last decade, service sector's contribution to the country's economy has been in the tune of over 50 per cent of GDP. The trend has been termed as 'India's Service Revolution' with rapid growth in the service industry. Particularly, education and healthcare are the key services, and a robust healthcare system would help create a strong human capital which in turn would result in higher productivity. Effective production, distribution and management of healthcare services is becoming increasingly important in order to make service operations profitable and meet the changing needs of people.

Healthcare industry is among the most rapidly growing services in the world economy, estimated at $4 trillion yearly in the OECD (Organization for Economic Co-operation and Development) countries alone. In the 1990s, the Indian healthcare industry grew at a compound annual rate of 16 per cent and is presently valued more than USD 34 billion roughly about 6 per cent of the Indian GDP. It is projected to reach USD 40 billion in the next few years. This sector has seen new and rapidly evolving forms that are spurred by wide-ranging factors such as technology, changing demographics, costs, skills, growing private sector participation, natural endowments, culture and geography (Chanda, 2005). The key objectives of an effective healthcare system are to enhance average life expectancy and to improve quality of life and productivity. The focus of healthcare industry is also moving from 'curing and treatment of diseases' to 'wellness'.

Healthcare Industry

The healthcare industry presents a very dynamic and uncertain environment. Continuous changes in technological, social, political, regulatory and economic contexts of healthcare delivery have made management of the organizations very challenging. Most countries including India, deliver healthcare services through a wide variety of network of public and private healthcare systems. It has emerged as one of the largest service sectors in India. Healthcare expenditure of a country is an important indicator of how well a country is equipped to meet the healthcare needs of its citizens. In 2004, national healthcare spending equalled about 5.2 per cent of the GDP and it is expected to rise by 13–15 per cent per annum through 2005–09 (in rupee terms) and scale up to about 5.5 per cent of the GDP by 2009 (IBEF, 2005). Other estimates suggest that by 2012, healthcare spending could contribute 8.5 per cent of the GDP and employ around nine million people (CII-McKinsey, 2002). Government share of the total expenditure is only 17 per cent, and therefore out-of-pocket expenditure is as high as 83 per cent. The private sector share is projected to be ₹ 1,600 billion, boosted by increasing penetration of health insurance. Health insurance is expected to generate a market spending of ₹ 400 billion in the healthcare services. However, India needs to add at least 80,000 beds each year to meet the growing demand for healthcare services, and to meet WHO norms on beds-to-population ratio. India's public health investment was 0.9 per cent of the GDP in 2001. Considering the needs of the people and the rising costs, the National Health

Policy, 2002 set a goal to increase health expenditure by the government from 0.9 to 2.0 per cent by the year 2010. The policy has further welcomed the participation of the private sector in all areas of healthcare activities – primary, secondary and tertiary in urban, rural and tribal areas (NHP, 2002). To bridge the demand-supply gap in healthcare services, it is estimated that an investment of nearly ₹ 100,000 to ₹ 140,000 crore is required (CII-McKinsey, 2002). Table 1 summarizes the market size and trends of the Indian healthcare industry.

Table 1.1

Indian Healthcare Industry: Market Size and Trends

<table>
<tr><th>Type of Services</th><th>Share of Healthcare Delivery Market (in %)</th><th>Health Expenditure % GDP*</th><td rowspan="2">Indian healthcare sector is expected to grow from US$ 18.7 billion to US$ 45 billion by 2010.</td></tr>
<tr><td>Primary, Secondary and Tertiary Care (All)</td><td>100</td><td>5.2 (Total)</td></tr>
<tr><td>Primary, Secondary and Tertiary Care (Public Sector)</td><td>37</td><td>0.9</td><td rowspan="2">Healthcare industry is estimated to grow from current 13% annually to 15% in the next 4–5 years.</td></tr>
<tr><td>Mostly Secondary and Tertiary (Private Sector)</td><td>63</td><td>4.3</td></tr>
</table>

Estimated Investments Needed in the Health Sector for the Next 10 Years

Investment	*Amount (₹ '000 Crore)*
Secondary Beds	60–90
Tertiary Beds	30–40
Medical Colleges	2–3
Nursing Schools	2–3
Other Health Professionals**	2–4
Total	100–140

Source: CII-McKinsey, 2002.

* World Development Report 2004, The World Bank.

** Pharmacists, technicians, administrators, etc.

The healthcare spending has been rising in many countries and the US healthcare expenditure is the highest among the industrialized nations. In 1999, the US spent about $4,000 per person annually on healthcare. The health expenses increased from 7.4 per cent of the GDP in 1970 to 13.6 per cent in 1996, and it is projected to reach 15.6 per cent by 2005 (Ginter et al., 2002). The US health expenditure is comparable with that of 9–10 per cent of Canada, France and Germany, and 6–7 per cent of Japan and the UK (Tabish, 1998). The expenditure incurred by the UK government on the National Health Service in 1992 was twice of that in 1984 (Aggarwal and Zairi, 1997). Rising costs of medical care is a major concern for most healthcare systems. Gaucher and Coffey (1993) concluded that all forms of new technology, ageing population, medical malpractice, overspecialization, the cost of poor quality, rework and waste, errors, variation in practice due to lack of standards and absence of incentives to control costs have resulted in rising healthcare costs.

Issues of funding, rising costs, utilization, consolidation, competition and quality along with political commitment dominated the healthcare sectors in the industrialized nations but in contrast a country like India struggles to increase its capacity to provide healthcare services to its huge population. The dynamic nature of the healthcare industry can be highlighted with two of the most researched health systems in the world, namely, that of the US and the National Health Service (NHS) of Great Britain. The US healthcare system has been identified as being costly and inefficient (Huq, 1996). In the UK at the end of 1970s, the NHS was at a crisis point and the universal healthcare as a basic right was in doubt. Recent reforms in the UK have produced an ideological and cultural hybrid of traditional public service values and business like orientation (Hewison, 2003). Major issues in the healthcare industry are that of consolidation of its service delivery in the US, advocating 'private healthcare delivery model' in the case of the UK and a need for huge investments and expansion in case of India.

Almost all countries undertake health sector reforms to serve their citizens and provide best possible healthcare. Peter Berman (1995, cited in Ramani and Mavalankar, 2005) described health sector reforms as "sustained, purposeful change to improve efficiency, equity, and effectiveness of the health sector. The implementation of large-scale health system reform demands political sensitivity, strategic thinking and management capacity of high order". In theory, the health sector reforms are meant to simultaneously promote equity and efficiency in the delivery of healthcare services, and to democratize the processes through which decisions about healthcare priorities are made. Health sector reforms are seen as a necessity to rationalize healthcare because the services available in a given setting often do not match the priority health needs of a population. In many countries, there has been proportionately more investment in secondary and tertiary care than in primary healthcare services. This has created stark regional disparities in the delivery of healthcare services. Moreover, weak infrastructure and inefficient use of resources inhibit delivery of good quality essential healthcare services. An increase in effectiveness of the healthcare system requires an efficient quality management system.

Quality Management in Healthcare Organizations

'Quality' is the central theme of all healthcare systems and is exceedingly becoming important for survival of healthcare organizations. In healthcare industry today, 'quality management' means not only patient recovery and satisfaction but also being cost effective for competitive advantage and survival. Quality in the context of healthcare services attains special significance due to the nature of the services which deals with life and death on a day-to-day basis. Chassin and Galvin (1998) have said that problems of healthcare quality are serious and extensive which occur in all healthcare delivery systems. The result is in terms of lost lives, reduced functioning and wasted resources. Quality in any sense is a comprehensive and multifaceted concept. Healthcare leaders are concerned about public accountability and consumerism that demand physical proof of efficiency and value. Quality has come to be recognized as a strategic tool for attaining operational efficiency and improved business performance (Jain and Gupta, 2004). Improving quality while reducing cost is not an easy task, but the organization's survival may depend on the managers' ability to do so. The focus of management of the majority of hospitals in India can be thought, in broad terms, as shifting from 'expansion' to 'quality for survival' in a competitive environment and finally to 'quality excellence' (Figure 1.1).

Figure 1.1
Focus of Management of Healthcare Organizations

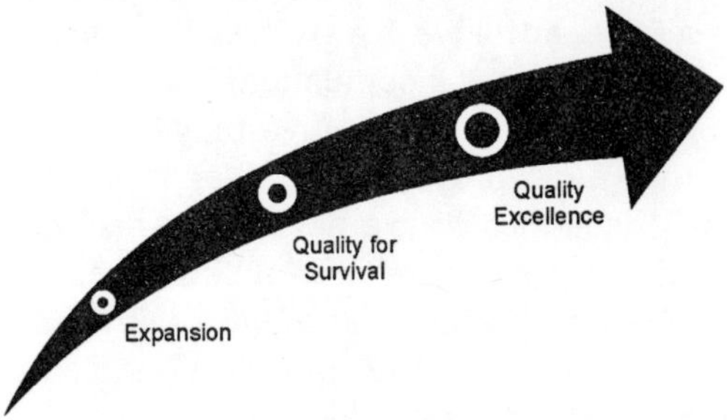

Fundamental approaches to managing quality at the organizational level can be broadly viewed under two categories, namely, Quality Assurance and Total Quality Management (also referred to as Continuous Quality Improvement, CQI). Quality Assurance (QA) involves regular external inspections to ensure that standards are being followed. The quality assurance mechanisms include different forms of external review such as accreditation, inspection, regulation, audit or external peer review (Potter et al., 1994; Walshe et al., 2001). BS 5750 and USA's Joint Commission on Accreditation of Healthcare Organizations (JCAHO) accreditation systems are examples of QA approaches. Another example is that of National Health Services (NHS) in England which uses the external review mechanisms very widely including medical training inspection, ISO 9000 quality management, external quality awards (such as 'Investors in People' and the Chartermark). Also, a number of accreditation schemes for many types of healthcare organizations exist (Thomson and Hodgson, 1997; Walshe et al., 2001). Accreditation is one of the most popular external mechanisms in healthcare. Further, accreditation as an external approach has been recommended as a mechanism of assuring the quality of private sector health services in low-income countries, especially where regulatory systems are weak (WHO, 1993). In India, Nandraj et al. (2001) examined the feasibility of introducing accreditation in Mumbai hospitals. The study demonstrated a provisional support of the hospital owners, professional bodies, government officials, consumer organizations and insurance/financial companies for accreditation. Accreditation in India (National Accreditation Board for Hospitals & Healthcare Organizations, NABH) is a new phenomenon and other regulatory mechanisms are quite weak. Though accreditation continues to be a very important mechanism of quality assurance, there is no consensus about standards or good practice and hence some conflicts between accreditation schemes do exist (Scrivens, 1995, cited in Hurst, 1997). The primary focus in accreditation is predominantly medical profession-based care management activities or controlling of adverse events. Though data-driven improvements in accreditation are emphasized, the evaluation requirements are relatively weak and benchmarking is lacking (Eggli and Halfon, 2003).

The majority of healthcare organizations use some form of audit methods to ensure quality of healthcare services. For instance, the healthcare reforms of NHS of the UK brought about progressive changes in the form of medical audit, clinical audit and clinical governance (Thomson and Hodgson, 1997; Brown and Bell, 1998). Integration of audit into routine clinical practice and hospital services is lacking in general. Another important quality management approach is that of ISO certification. In the recent years, many hospitals in India have obtained ISO certification to indicate the hospital's commitment to quality. However, ISO does not focus on what should be improved in an organization in order to gain competitive position. In general, ISO certification focuses on the documentation of management systems and on the consistency in the production of a product or a service, and provides a common basis for assuring buyers that specific practices are in conformance with the provider's stated quality systems (Zhu and Scheuermann, 1999). A number of studies have shown that ISO certification is more static and has limited focus on people and continuous improvement (Low, 1998; Hind, 1996; Priebe, 2000; Eggli and Halfon, 2003; Magd and Curry, 2003; Tari, 2005). Further, the development of ISO is driven by the existing users but most of them are not related to healthcare. Industry leaders in India are also voicing their concerns about the usefulness of ISO and JCAHO certification for Indian hospitals (Viswanathan, 2002a). Based on their study on external reviews on quality in healthcare organizations, Walshe et al. (2001) concluded that external reviews rarely generate wholly new knowledge and are not revelatory, and hence do not usually lead to major changes in policy, strategy or practice. The studies indicate that to improve quality and competitiveness, the logical next step for organizations would be the use of a Total Quality Management (TQM) model involving customer-focus, key-process monitoring, data-driven tools and techniques and team empowerment.

Emergence of Total Quality Management in Healthcare

Traditionally, healthcare services have been provider centric with professionals making major decisions about what is good for the patients owing to their technical knowledge and expertise. In general, today's healthcare organizations function on values built early on in the 20th century and lag behind changes that are seen in service settings, service designs and relationships between provider and client in non-healthcare sector. Contributions of the quality gurus namely, Deming, Juran, Crosby, Feigenbaum and Ishikawa have had a great impact on the quality management in manufacturing and service industries. Similarly, the works of Donabedian, Berwick, Bluementhal, Kazandjian, McLaughlin, Kaluzny and others are of great interest to healthcare quality management. A new way of thinking in terms of evidence-based medicine, health technology assessment, customer orientation and cost effective services are on the quality agenda of every healthcare professional (Øvretveit, 1997).

Operationalization of the concepts of quality at the organizational level has led to several innovations in quality management, from traditional quality assurance to implementation of the philosophy of TQM. "Under the ever-increasing pressure to contain costs while maintaining or improving quality of care, the market place has become an increasingly unfamiliar, uncertain, and unfriendly environment for hospitals, many are turning to different sources for help. While the TQM philosophy has its roots in manufacturing and industry, it is based on many techniques, which could easily be transferred to the health care setting. Actually, the medical field has some advantages over the manufacturing sector. These include: familiarity with statistical methods, a mentality to seek continuous improvement in care and the ability to work in teams as a routine practice" (Huq, 1996, p. 59). TQM is a new approach to quality improvement and it encompasses all systems and processes, clinical and non-clinical, with actions directed towards processes to improve the quality of all services and products for customers (Gaucher and Coffey, 1993, p. 20). TQM is not a quick fix and rewards come after a number of years, but it helps to build a culture of quality among employees, involves everyone and is progressive. The realization that it is possible to increase quality and reduce cost by nearly 30 per cent in a service industry by eliminating waste, duplication and non-value added cost, and thereby improving customer satisfaction, customer retention and profits, has underpinned successive quality drives in service industries in the US (Reichheld and Sasser, 1990; Caldwell, 1997). Total quality revolution has perhaps been considered very influential and pervasive among management initiatives in healthcare organizations worldwide over the past few years (Adinolfi, 2003). Kazandjian (1997a, p. 2) puts it this way 'In the pursuit of ongoing improvement of performance "zero error", "optimal production efficiency" and "hundred per cent appropriateness" have become the de facto limits'.

TQM is a quality-oriented approach that consists of applying a selection of quality management techniques throughout the organization with the aim to achieve overall organizational goals and objectives through customer focus. It gives a healthcare organization an opportunity for a higher level of competitiveness over a period of time. Many studies in healthcare have shown a number of advantages of implementation of TQM in quality of services, customer satisfaction, perceptions of quality, earnings, improved outcomes, etc. (Gaucher and Coffey, 1993; Klein et al., 1995; Anderson et al., 1996; Moody et al., 1998; Klein et al., 1998; Bharat et al., 1999; McLaughlin and Simpson, 1999; Singhal et al., 2000; Chow-Chua and Goh, 2002; Chang and Cheng, 2003). Based on empirical research on the success parameters for quality management and business performance in hospitals, Kunst and Lemmink (2000) concluded that the progress in TQM leads to higher business performance (indicating efficiency), and a higher perceived service quality by patients (indicating effectiveness). Short and Rahim (1995) have said that the traditional focus of technical quality inherent in healthcare can be extended to include overall services to achieve excellence through adaptation of TQM principles. For effective implementation of TQM in an organization, it is important to identify critical quality management strategies. Such 'critical success factors or strategies' correspond to the drivers of quality performance (Kanji and SÁ, 2003). Operational measures of quality management in terms of certain critical factors would be useful to both decision-makers and researchers. Decision-makers need to know the status and level of variables of quality management that can be effectively controlled in order to achieve high quality. The researchers can use such measures to understand quality management practice much better and build theories and models on quality management. Usefulness of quality models is two-fold: one, for measurement of quality levels of organizations and two, for implementation of quality management strategies in an integrated manner for continuous improvement.

Figure 1.2
Broad Classifications of Quality Management Methods

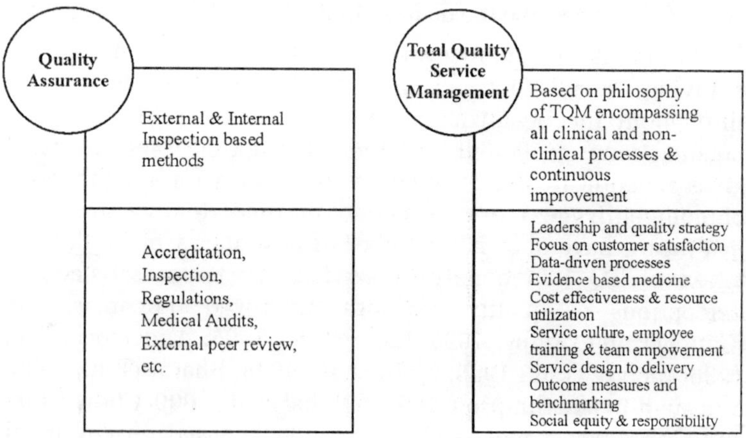

Critical factor research on TQM can be approached from various methods: studying from quality leaders, formal evaluation models (e.g., MBNQA) and empirical research.

Critical Factors for TQM Implementation

Research on critical success factors for TQM implementation in non-healthcare context is quite well established (Saraph et al., 1989; Ahire et al., 1996; Black and Porter, 1996; Ang et al., 2000; Zhang et al., 2000). Researchers have often used Baldrige framework, as it is comprehensive and used by many organizations (Black and Porter, 1996; Flynn and Saladin, 2001; Sila and Ebrahimpour, 2003). Counte and Meurer (2001) analysed the current measures and studies of CQI implementation in healthcare organizations worldwide. The results of the study indicated that there is a need for more research on increased use of criteria other than the Baldrige categories, increased focus on financial variables, improved measures of implementation stage and the use of different types of respondents from multiple organization levels. In general, top management commitment and leadership, customer focus, information and analysis, training, supplier management, process management, teamwork, product and service design, process control, benchmarking, continuous improvement, employee empowerment, quality assurance, social responsibility and employee satisfaction are the most commonly extracted factors in many of the studies. Consensus on criticality of factors of TQM across nations is difficult, though generic models have been very useful in understanding intricacies of TQM implementation. External business contexts in terms of the country's economic and social development, culture, religion, education levels, information technology, government regulations, the extent of industrialization and TQM maturity levels are known to affect the criticality of the factors for successful TQM implementation (Lakhe and Mohanty, 1994; Tari, 2002; Sila and Ebrahimpour, 2003; Mohanty and Lakhe, 2006). Therefore, there is a need for researchers to evaluate the applicability of a generic model developed and validated in a country such as USA to a developing country such as India. In fact, many researchers have identified the need for investigation of critical factors for successful implementation of TQM in hospitals. Such a research with inputs from senior hospitals managers from a large number of organizations would be very fruitful for arriving at a model for Total Quality Services (TQS) in the sector (Lin and Clousing, 1995; Adinolfi, 2003; Øvretveit and Gustafson, 2003; Sila and Ebrahimpour, 2003).

Services, more so healthcare services, are intangible in nature. It is well known that aspects of service intangibility, simultaneity of production, delivery and consumption, perishability, variability of expectations of customers and participatory role of customers in the service delivery render the transportability of quality management practices of manufacturing to the healthcare sector rather difficult. Parasuraman et al. (1985, 1988) identified and developed measuring instrument (SERVQUAL) for services quality with five dimensions, namely, tangibility, reliability, responsiveness, assurance and empathy. However, the validity and reliability of the dimensions are debatable (Cuganeshan et al., 1997). Also, SERVQUAL is limited in its approach and does not specifically address the important dimensions of QM such as top management commitment, staff focus, training and development for continuous improvement, measurement and analysis of quality data, supplier quality issues, etc. Sureshchandar et al. (2001a, b) developed a holistic model for TQS and empirically validated the model using the survey method in the banking sector in India. Their model included service culture and servicescapes as important criteria for service sector and the importance of those factors in healthcare services is obvious. They recommended that the instrument could be used with necessary modifications for healthcare and other service organizations. Healthcare-specific elements such as epidemiological studies, medical records data, involvement of the medical staff governance process (quality assurance methods such as peer review, hospital acquired infection committee, audit committee), risk-adjusted outcome measures (based on severity of illness, age, etc.), cost-effective analysis, use of quality assurance data and risk-management data may have to be incorporated in TQM of hospitals (McLaughlin and Kaluzny, 1999, pp. 8–10). In healthcare settings, Huq (1996) arrived at a framework of TQM dimensions based on the works of the quality gurus and it includes management control and implementation issues in TQM. However, rigorous statistical methodology for theory building was not reported in the study and a measurement instrument was not fully developed. Quality award criteria (EQA and MBNQA) are often used as a basis for TQM implementation in hospitals. However, investigating on the relationship between quality and business performance of hospitals in three European countries, Kunst and Lemmink (2000) concluded that the general application of European Quality Award Criteria (based on European Foundation for Quality Management, EFQM) as an evaluation instrument is debatable. Considering the specific needs of healthcare, MBNQA in 1999 came up with criteria for hospital services. Meyer and Collier (2001) empirically tested the causal relationships in the Baldrige Health Care Pilot Criteria and this is one of the comprehensive researches that validated the criteria for TQM implementation in healthcare. It needs to be evaluated for the Indian context. Further, Chow-Chua and Goh (2002) presented a model which integrated Singapore Quality Award criteria (similar to Baldrige criteria) and the balanced score card (BSC) approach. Kanji and SÁ (2003) presented an implementation and measurement model to help sustain healthcare excellence; however they did not empirically validate the model. The above discussion indicates that more research is needed for validating the criteria for total quality in healthcare.

In the Indian context, professional management of hospitals has increasingly gaining importance since the 1990s, but research on TQS is very limited. Studies on implementation of quality management strategies such as process management (Varghese, 2001; Reddy and Acharyulu, 2003), patient satisfaction/expectation surveys (Bhardwaj et al., 2001; Mahapatra et al., 2001; Verma and Sobti, 2002), reducing hospital infection rates (Vij et al., 2001; Gupta, 2004) and TQM in various hospital departments (Reddy et al., 2002; Arya et al., 2003) are reported. However, organization-wide implementation is a new phenomenon. At the hospital level, Tata Main Hospital, Jamshedpur, India, has implemented TQM. Tata Business Excellence Model (TBEM) based on MBNQA criteria, formed the basis of the hospital's TQM implementation (Bharat, 2001). In general, the quality of care among

Indian hospitals varies quite considerably and in the absence of proper regulatory and accreditation mechanisms, it is difficult to accurately judge the quality levels of the hospitals (Nandraj et al., 2001). The hospitals are beginning to formalize quality management practices in order to provide high quality services. Research in this area would provide hospital managers with specific guidelines and directions for quality management strategies in the Indian context. Therefore, to fill the research gap, this study proposed to develop an integrative framework of critical success factors of the TQM principles for achieving TQS in healthcare organizations.

Overview of the Chapters

Many hospitals in India are now concentrating on improving the quality of healthcare services in order to succeed in the competitive market. A comprehensive study would be useful to understand the factors critical to successful implementation of Total Quality Service Management in the hospital sector. Such a research was taken up and an integrative framework for TQS for the sector was developed based on extensive literature survey and analysis, expert inputs and cross-sectional survey of hospitals. Rigorous qualitative and quantitative research analysis was applied to ensure reliability and reliability of the TQS framework.

Following this introductory chapter where background and broad objectives of the research are presented, there are nine more chapters. A brief description of these nine chapters is given here.

Chapter 2 on Core Issues in Healthcare Quality presents an analysis of need for quality initiatives and reforms and core issues in healthcare. The issues of process and outcome quality, freedom from deficiencies and features of services, quality in fact and quality in perception are discussed. The chapter concludes that healthcare managers could consider 'quality as a construct' with various dimensions and stakeholder interests and ensure that all these dimensions are addressed adequately in quality management programmes.

Chapter 3 on Quality Assurance in Healthcare closely examines accreditation, medical audits and ISO approaches. Their applications and limitations are critically assessed. Given the market realities of competition, globalization and consumer awareness, most of all technological and management advances, healthcare organizations have to move from inspection-oriented quality improvement system to one that orients itself to a systematic transformation of organizational culture through a comprehensive plan involving customer focus, key-process monitoring, data-driven tools and techniques, and team empowerment. The chapter concludes that the philosophy and operationalization of TQM techniques for healthcare would be the choice of methods for healthcare managers.

Chapter 4 on Total Quality Management in Healthcare reviews the literature on the concepts, issues, advantages, applications and general framework of TQM in healthcare. The contributions of 'Quality Gurus' such as Deming, Juran, Feigenbaum, Crosby and Ishikawa in general are briefly discussed and specific contributions of healthcare quality by Donabedian, Berwick, McGlaughlin, Kaluzny and Simpson are closely examined. The chapter traces how managing total quality of healthcare services is gaining ground in the hospital sector. Finally, the case of TQM for healthcare organizations as very useful for achieving sustainable improvements in quality, processes enhancements and cost advantages based on philosophical, structural and healthcare elements of Total Quality Services Management is established.

Chapter 5 on Quality Management of Healthcare Services in India discusses the quality issues, challenges and initiatives by the health sector in India. In general, regulatory mechanisms in India are quite weak and accreditation schemes for hospitals are an emerging area. Based on literature review, it is found that measurement of results of hospital-wide TQM applications is very limited and research in the area of critical success factors for TQS is lacking in our country. This supports the view that research on development of Total Quality Service framework is very useful.

Chapter 6 on Research on Quality Dimensions for TQS Implementation presents literature analysis of several quality management models and frameworks from literature to identify the critical quality dimensions. Barriers to TQM implementation in hospitals, research on perceived service quality, quality award criteria, TQM critical factors research from manufacturing, services and healthcare research are reviewed. A 13-construct Total Quality Service (TQS) framework with associated scales that accurately captures the TQS criteria specifically for hospitals is identified.

Chapter 7 on Validating Quality Constructs: Observations from Studies in Indian Hospitals presents two empirical research studies for content validation of TQS constructs: one, quality performance measurement of a case hospital using MBNQA healthcare criteria and two, qualitative analysis of survey of Quality Management practices among Indian hospitals. The studies provided support to the appropriateness of the 13-construct TQS framework and are useful in improvising the measuring instrument for TQS.

Chapter 8 on Empirical Investigation on TQS presents the results and discussion of the testing and analysis of the TQS measuring instrument with 118 items grouped appropriately as 13 quality constructs. Survey results of the research on the TQS constructs involving senior managers from major hospitals in India and statistical analysis for reliability and validity as well as confirmatory factor analysis are presented. Discussions highlight the insights from the Indian hospital sector.

Chapter 9 on Integrative Framework for Total Quality Service Management in Hospitals presents the relationship among 13 TQS constructs. Various tested TQM models for services and healthcare are analysed and relationships among the criteria are synthesized. A conceptual integrative framework for TQS management for hospitals consisting of Driver, Enabler and Goals as holistic and interrelated systems is arrived at. It is suggested that the hospitals could use TQS Index for assessing their quality levels and make decisions about further improvements in quality of services.

Chapter 10 on Conclusions and Future Research Directions summarizes the entire research work and identifies the limitations of the study and future directions for research in the area of Total Quality Service for healthcare. Research based on literature analysis, academic, field expert and practitioner inputs would continue to improve the understanding (and hence implementation) of criticality and nuances of TQS in hospitals.

2

Core Issues in Healthcare Quality

Challenges in managing a healthcare organization in the present context and limitations of the existing mechanisms for quality management have resulted in innovative methods to manage quality. The motivation for improving quality is economic as well as a strategy for organizations. Pursuit of quality would maximize effective and efficient care as well as reduce waste and ineffectiveness. Many hospitals, clinics, healthcare organizations, private companies and health systems have launched initiatives to reduce medical errors, improve patient safety, patient satisfaction and quality of care. While defining quality of care, it is important to differentiate between 'medical services' and 'healthcare services'. Services that a qualified physician determines for assessment, prevention, treatment, rehabilitation or palliation of a given health problem based on professional experience and consensus and/or available scientific evidence could be thought of as 'medical services'. Healthcare services are services provided not only by (or under supervision of) physicians but also those wide range of services performed by healthcare professionals such as nurses, physiotherapists, health educators, nutritionists, psychologists, dentists and so on. Frameworks for quality at micro level (individual practitioner level), meso level (organization level) and macro level (health systems level) are very useful tools to initiate quality initiatives. This work focuses on the 'meso level' quality management of healthcare services and takes into consideration the needs of multiple stakeholders involved to achieve 'total quality'. But then, what is 'quality'?

Concepts of quality in healthcare are a much debated topic. However, quality initiatives and concepts are obviously not new to healthcare. In the field of medicine, quality of care has always been important and medical professionals take oath to provide quality of care. The roots of quality assurance initiatives in health care extend at least as far back as the time of Florence Nightingale's work during the Crimean war (1854–56), when the introduction of nutrition, sanitation and infection control initiatives in war hospitals contributed to a reduction in the death rate from 43 to 2 per cent (cited in Mohanty et al., 1996). She developed and used a systematic approach to collecting and analysing information on differences in mortality rates. Perhaps Ernest Codman may be considered as the first physician to advocate TQM for hospitals. In 1910, in the, Ernest Codman, M.D., (1869–1940), Surgeon, Massachusetts General Hospital, Harvard Medical School proposed the 'end result system of hospital standardization'. Under this system, a hospital would track every patient it treated long enough to determine whether the treatment was effective (Codman, 1910 cited in DesHarnais and McLaughlin, 1999, pp. 59–60). If the treatment was not effective, the hospital would then attempt to determine why, so that similar cases could be treated successfully in future.

Need for Quality Initiatives

In the present context, the reasons for countries around the world to improve the quality of healthcare have been related to issues of funding the ever growing costs of healthcare, utilization, consolidation, competition, equity, regulations, changing spectrum of epidemiology of diseases, demographic changes and so on. The greatest challenges facing the service organizations today are the ever-growing competition and the continuous increase in customer expectations (Coddington et al., 1985; Kumar et al., 1997; Kandampully and Butler, 2001). The challenges for providing cost-effective high-quality care among industrialized nations are given in Figure 2.1. The following section examines the reasons for quality initiatives and reforms in healthcare systems across the world.

Figure 2.1

Challenges for the Industrialized Nations in Healthcare Quality Management

Dramatic increases in life expectancies- about three years per decade, and the aging of the general population.

Success of biomedical research, resulting in a doubling of medical knowledge about every four years.

Rapid diffusion of expensive high tech medical procedures into daily practice.

Transformation of the epidemiological spectrum, characterized by the decline of acute infectious diseases and the growing importance of chronic illnesses

Source: Köeck (1997) in his foreword to the book 'The Effectiveness of CQI in Health Care: Stories from a Global Perspective' stresses that the healthcare systems of industrialized nations are undergoing dramatic and rapid changes.

Reasons for Quality Initiatives and Reforms in Healthcare

Particular characteristics of each healthcare system differ from country to country, and each system develops mechanisms to cope with internal (organizational) and external environmental challenges. As one would expect, there are underlying common features in those challenges, which indicate that some problems are similar across nations and some are unique to a particular healthcare delivery system.

1. *Issues of rising costs of healthcare* have dominated almost all health systems including the industrialized nations. In general, ageing population, costs-of- and possible overuse-of-advanced technologies, medical malpractice,

costs of poor quality, rework and waste, errors, variations in practice due to lack of standards and absence of incentives to control costs have resulted in higher healthcare costs (Gaucher and Coffey, 1993, pp. 9–16). Such cost issues led to a large number of failures, mergers and alliances in the US (Huq, 1996; Ginter et al., 2002) and in the UK the NHS debated on reforms and costs of quality (Thomson and Hodgson, 1997). Therefore, there is an ever-growing need for innovative ways to provide quality care at reduced costs.

2. *Increased public knowledge and expectations* has led to concerns regarding waiting time especially for non-emergency surgical treatment, amenity and interpersonal aspects of care, medical consumerism (both in lobbying and actions of consumer advocacy groups, consumers' concerns on value and demands for accountability and efficiency. This in turn has made service providers and hospitals develop inclusive quality frameworks.
3. *Variations in clinical practice, errors and adverse events* in healthcare services understandably have provoked media, public, provider and purchaser interest in improving the delivery processes (Boyce, 1997; Buchan, 1998; Weingart et al., 2000; Kazandjian, 2004). A report from the Institute of Medicine, USA, states that around 100,000 patients per year die from preventable errors in hospitals in the US (Editor's Choice, BMJ, 2000). Involvement of physicians, evidence-based medicine, benchmarking, data-based comparisons and training in clinical and non-clinical processes and process improvements have become crucial to quality management (Berwick et al., 1990, pp. 145–157 cited in McLaughlin and Simpson, 1999, pp. 34–35).
4. *Stifling bureaucratic management structures* in hospitals have resulted in inefficiencies, wastefulness and remoteness from those served. Further, they are known to adversely affect staff motivation and implementation of new procedures. Decentralization and reorganization in order to achieve better patient and employee satisfaction are being considered by the organizations.
5. *Transition in the epidemiological profile* including the demographic profile of growing elderly population is

common in many countries. In addition, infectious diseases have been brought under control but chronic illnesses and injuries have increased in frequency. Emergent problems such as AIDS and diverse health effects from environmental pollution as well as resurgent problems such as cholera have resulted in a competition for resources.

6. *External imperatives and regulations from government, purchasers and regulatory agencies* to monitor quality of healthcare services have led to the development of relevant quality indicators (Boyce, 1997). Hospitals are sincerely putting quality assurance programmes in place, for instance NABH implementation by many hospitals in India.
7. *Cost containment and competition* have been a major theme underlying quality initiatives in many cases. Hospital managers are extremely becoming 'quality conscious' and in fact, 'quality and affordability' have become the mantra for hospitals in India to achieve the competitive edge in the fast growing sector.

Short and Rahim (1995) have pointed out that the problem of hospitals is further compounded by decreasing funding and services utilization, and increasing consolidation and competition. "The pressure to change has been driven by escalating costs and increased demands from both dissatisfied patients and third party payers. A movement that holds great promise for improved health care quality and productivity is the introduction of TQM. Spurred by impressive results in other industries, this compelling and logical approach has begun to penetrate the thinking of health care accrediting agencies, private foundations and leading health care organizations." In order to achieve excellence in quality of healthcare, 'quality' needs to be defined in clear terms.

Core Issues in Defining Healthcare Quality

Quality means different things to different people. All of us would intuitively know what quality is but may not be able to clearly define it. In healthcare, it is obvious that a patient would include 'getting well' or 'cured' as one important criterion for judging the quality of the service. However, it is often debated whether the patient will be able to judge the technical aspects of the medical care appropriately because of the specialized nature of medical knowledge. In general, the professional viewpoint as to what and how of quality has dominated the debate in healthcare services (Figure 2.2).

Figure 2.2
Core Issues in Healthcare Quality

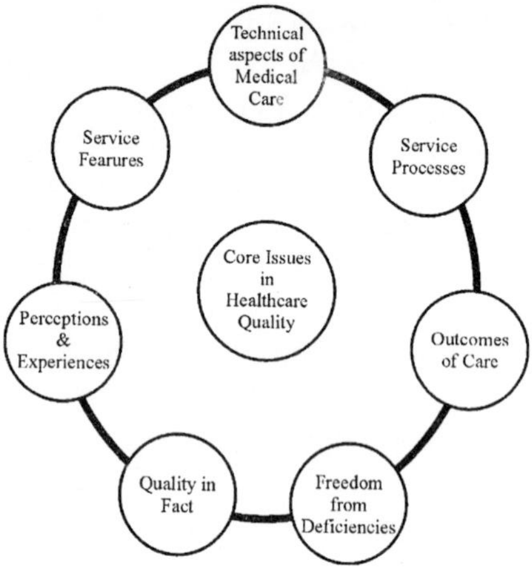

Technical Aspects of Healthcare Quality: 'All about Medical Care'

Traditionally, quality of care is considered primarily dependent on provider knowledge and meeting professional standards. Quality is inherent in the professional standards, guidelines, codes of the myriad of professions involved in healthcare, and associations that represent these professionals and the healthcare organizations themselves. Medical errors and patient safety continues to be a major concern for all involved in providing high quality clinical care (Sutcliffe, 2004). The Joint Commission on Accreditation of Healthcare Organizations (JCAHO) of the USA and the National Committee for Quality Assurance have stimulated interest in developing quality measures. The challenges are:

1. To always provide effective care to those who could benefit from it.

2. To always refrain from providing inappropriate services.
3. To eliminate all preventable complications.

As participant observers of the National Roundtable on Health Care Quality, Chassin and Galvin (1998) have classified the problems of healthcare into three categories: underuse (missing measles vaccine), overuse (potential harm exceeds its potential benefits) and misuse (preventable complication occurs after an appropriate medical procedure).

In general, the quality of care means comparing actual properties of care with professional requirements and with expectations of patients or the society. Institute of Medicine, in its seminal 2001 report, *Crossing the Quality Chasm: A New Health System for the 21st Century,* defined quality as: "Quality of care is the degree to which health services for individuals and populations increase the likelihood of desired health outcomes and are consistent with current professional knowledge" (cited in Goonan, 1995, p. 15). The definition includes two important concepts: measurement and knowledge. Experts continue to work to create reliable and valid measures with which to assess the quality of healthcare over a wide range of diagnostic and therapeutic services and for a broad array of health and medical problems.

It is often argued that on one hand, defining quality of care from the physician perspective alone has limitations and on the other, non-provider customers (e.g., patients) are not competent to judge technical and scientific quality (Gaucher and Coffey, 1993). Most measures of quality are indicative of quality or process failure, e.g., mortality, morbidity, hospital-acquired infection rates and unplanned readmissions. These measures are neither customer focused nor focused on excellence. There would be few patients who would go to a hospital expecting any of these complications to occur. Further, the concept of quality gets more complex looking at the traditional view that "quality means doing more" – using greater technology, doing more tests, giving more intensive care, etc. Development of Clinical Practice Guidelines (CPGs) containing relevant clinical recommendations based on scientific evidence (concept of Evidence Based Medicine), consensus of experts and experienced practitioners has been a major trend to reduce variations in practice and promote EBM. For example, preventive care recommends mammography screening among women 50–59 years of age.

However, most of the physicians have problems accepting fundamental challenges such as 'patients are well equipped to assess core dimensions of the quality of care they receive'. The knowledge differential between physicians and patients is obvious. But chronic illnesses are becoming more prevalent and the patient has to assume the functions traditionally reserved for the provider of the care, e.g., diabetes or heart disease cannot be treated in an organized manner effectively and efficiently without the patient's participation. Therefore, understanding patient preferences should become foundations of organizations and hence an important quality dimension in addition to technical quality (Köeck, 1997).

Process and Outcome Quality: 'Service Processes and Outcomes'

One area that causes considerable difficulty in the service sector is the confusion that exists between *process quality* and *outcome quality*. Outcome quality is often wholly dependent on the specialists or consultants, this we have already examined under technical aspects of quality. But process quality depends on support processes that are not necessarily provided only by physicians. The clients or patients will be evaluating the process quality as part of the whole experience of healthcare service. Macdonald (1994) gives the following example to highlight the differences in process and outcome quality:

For a patient entering a hospital for surgery:

1. Process quality is:
    - Admissions and ward staff friendly, responsive and professional
    - Ward quiet, clean and well equipped with patient-oriented service as well as technical equipment
    - Food good and sufficient
    - Visitor relations handled well

2. Outcome quality is:
   - Patient's recovery
   - Minimal after-effects
   - Wounds healing quickly

Outcomes are not always easy to measure (like in clinical trials) in healthcare. With the focus on hospital care, the quality of outcome, hospital care, and physician care are all modelled as components of overall quality of care. The relative importance of the technical dimension of hospital care, such as outcome of physician care and nursing care (i.e., is the patient free from the disease, pain or incapacity that had caused the hospitalization?) versus the affective dimensions (e.g., food, noise, room temperature, privacy and parking) have been a source of tension among physicians, hospital managers and health plans. Patients will focus on health gains, satisfaction or well being on the one hand, and wants, needs and expectations on the other. The medical professional will judge the effect of medical interventions against a background of scientific knowledge, whereas the manager of hospitals will focus on the costs and the number of interventions delivered in relation to the available materials and manpower. All three groups of people judge quality in the same way but differ in their focus on specific aspects of medical care on the one hand and in their expectations on the other (Harteloh, 2003). Hospital and health-plan marketeers argue that customers evaluate the quality of processes, namely, the personal service they receive and the accommodation amenities of the hospital, and that the customer is always right.

The US Office of Technology Assessment has defined the quality of care as "the degree to which the process of care increases the probability of outcomes desired by the patient, and reduces the probability of undesired outcomes, given the state of medical knowledge" (U.S. Congress of Technology Assessment, 1988, cited in DesHarnais and McLaughlin, 1999, p. 66). Though the definition relates processes, outcomes and patients accurately, measurement and relations of all is difficult if not impossible. Measurement of data from healthcare processes displays a natural variation which can be modeled using a variety of statistical distributions. Use of control charts (tools of Statistical Process Control, SPC), for instance, can often yield insights into data more quickly and is easy to use for decision-making than traditional statistical methods. For example, control charts for flash sterilization rate, laboratory turnaround time, surgical site infections, appointment access satisfaction, infectious waste monitoring, etc. can be used to study variations and improvements after specific intervention techniques (Benneyan et al., 2003).

Freedom from Deficiencies and Features: 'Errors and Service Features'

One definition that has proved useful in many quality management programmes includes two simple concepts: freedom from deficiencies and features (Goonan, 1995). Deficiencies occur in almost all organizations and professions, and healthcare is no exception. When processes and people fail to achieve optimal results, they create potentially preventable patient suffering, wasted resources, unnecessary work for colleagues and in some cases risk of litigation. A clinical process deficiency can be defined as any avoidable error or unnecessary step in prevention, diagnosis and treatment of a health problem. Some examples of deficiencies include the following: the time and resources that go into unnecessary care; the absence of necessary care; wasted resources such as blood products or drugs; preventable complications; days in an acute-care hospital waiting for bed; practice patterns that deviate from recognized guidelines; nosocomial infections; ER triage delays, unplanned return to surgery; post-operative arrhythmia and lost lab results. Deficiencies when known to patients, lead to dissatisfaction, distrust and diminished loyalty. On the other hand, the absence of deficiencies does not necessarily lead to increased patient loyalty. When deficient care receives publicity, the loss of market share and reputation can be tremendous. Features are defined as the aspects of patient care that attract patients, that distinguish one practitioner from another or one hospital care from others (such as unsolicited phone calls to the patient or family, evening and weekend hours, patient education videos, patient reminder cards, etc.). Features are not necessary for optimal care but patients may seek and value certain ones (Goonan, 1995). This market-based approach is rather easy to implement and may have immediate impact on 'perceptions' though may indirectly increase the costs.

Quality in Fact and Quality in Perception: 'Measurement and Experiences'

Another important set of concepts useful in judging quality in healthcare is 'quality in fact' and 'quality in perception'. Researchers and quality assurance experts have made significant efforts to find valid and reliable measures of quality, cost, performance, outcomes and satisfaction, e.g., use of complication rates and procedural appropriateness rates (Joint Commission, 1990, cited in Goonan, 1995, pp. 20–23). Survey methodologies have evolved and can be considered as another objective source of reporting on certain patient-care experiences. In general, patients are viewed as a source of perceptual but not factual information about healthcare experience (Collingwood, 1996). Perceptions definitely play a major role in physician, hospital and healthcare procedure or plan selection. Reputation of the hospital, anecdote, expert opinion and personal reference are a part of quality in perception, e.g., patients can be an accurate source of information about what procedures they have had or whether they understand how to take their medications. Such information can be measured by patient reports through surveys, interviews, focus groups, etc. Other sources for factual measurement of quality are the medical records and administrative databases. In addition, development of SERVQUAL for measuring 'perceived service quality' on five dimensions (tangibles, reliability, responsiveness, assurance and empathy) by Parasuraman et al. (1985, 1988) can be useful in healthcare.

Study by Carman provides new insights into whether patients can assess technical aspects of quality (facts) and perceptual aspects of quality. Carman (2000) studied how patients evaluate the quality of hospital care. Using conjoint methodology, Carman empirically investigated and found that technical dimensions of nursing care, physician care and outcomes are more important than the accommodation functions of hospital care. However, both sets of dimensions emerged important and significant. It was found that patients were able to evaluate technical and affective (emotion based) components separately, and affective components did not essentially influence technical quality evaluations.

Quality as a Construct

From management perspective, integrating the above concepts of medical and technical care (physician perspective), service levels and features (patient perspective), operational ease and cost effectiveness (manager's perspective), and measurement and evidence (scientific perspective) have to be modeled into developing 'Quality as a Construct'. The above discussion leads to three main components of quality, namely, Technical Quality, Administrative Quality and Service Quality.

Let us consider three levels of quality as given by Dumas et al., 1987 (cited in McLaughlin and Kaluzny, 1999, p. 31):

1. *Conformance quality* is conforming to specifications; having a product or service that meets predetermined standards.
2. *Requirements quality* means meeting total customer requirements; having perceived attributes of a service or product that meet or exceed customer requirements.
3. *Quality in kind* refers to extraordinary quality that delights the customer; having perceived attributes of a product or service that significantly exceed customer expectations, thereby delighting the customer with its value.

Priebe (2000) emphasizes that a way out of the dilemma to find a universally valid definition of quality may be deduced by radical constructivism. According to this philosophy, quality can be seen as a construct. Constructs are maintained, modified or given up not because they are true or false, but because they are more or less useful to the one holding them. The usefulness of a construct depends on the perspective and the interests of the individual stakeholder. All the interests are legitimate, but are likely to be associated with different priorities for quality assurance and quality improvement. This perspective of radical constructivism helps to understand why there is no overall accepted and eternal definition of quality and no single 'right approach' for ensuring and improving it. The most important message is that it is a philosophy of change and a comprehensive exercise involving all levels of the healthcare system, and not just a mere technique to be applied through external pressure. This means that healthcare managers can consider quality as a construct with various dimensions and ensure that all these dimensions are addressed adequately in quality management programmes. Such a viewpoint would lead quality of care to include the technical aspects of care processes (and outcomes), administrative processes and service aspects of care (reflected as perceptions and satisfaction by patients, families, etc.).

Considering the core issues discussed above, quality management programmes of hospitals have to ensure the following elements of quality (Figure 2.3):

Figure 2.3

Modelling Core Issues of Quality into Management Programme

Appropriateness	• Was treatement necessary? • Was it the right treatement?
Competence	• Are doctors knowledge and skills appropriate? • Are they regularly monitored, retrained and licensed?
Technical Performance	• Did the treatments/procedures adhere to standards? • Were the tasks performed by health workers as per expectations?
Safety	• Are potential risks minimized or avoided? • Do patients know about the procedures and understand care procedures?
Effectiveness of care	• Did the treatment procedures result in positive outcomes? • Has the patient survival and quality of life improved?
Efficiency of service delivery	• Were resource utilization minimized (tests, materials, equipment, time, facilities, etc.)? Were procedures and processes streamlined?
Acceptability	• Were the expectations of the patients and family met? • Were the treatment procedures carried out as per referring doctor's orders?
Access to services	• Is the facility accessiible to patients? • Were the services provided in a timely manner?
Interpersonal relations and choice	• Is the trust, respect, courtesy and empathy reflected in communication and interactions? • Is choice of the patient for treatment procedures and specialisits considered?
Physical infrastructure and comfort	• Facility cleanliness and aesthetics conducive to well being and recovery? • Is technology and equipment properly set?

The above model includes the features that form the core of healthcare quality. The framework helps healthcare professionals to define, analyse and measure programme standards for clinical care and services that support service delivery. The implementation model has to define quality in clear terms, establish implementation plan and measure the outcomes of care processes. In general, quality management in hospitals and healthcare organizations are based on the use of a number of quality assurance (QA) mechanisms (Manjunath, 2008). The next chapter examines the most commonly used QA mechanisms and analyses the limitations of such mechanisms in addressing total quality issues of healthcare services.

Summary

Quality in any sense is a comprehensive and multifaceted concept. Traditionally, healthcare services have been provider-centric with professionals making major decisions about what is good for the patients owing to technical knowledge and expertise. This chapter discussed the core issues involved in defining healthcare quality. Since quality has come to be recognized as a strategic tool for attaining operational efficiency and improved business performance of healthcare organizations, healthcare managers need to arrive at a more comprehensive definition of healthcare quality. Issues of technical aspects of quality as well as process and outcome quality, quality in fact and perception, and freedom from deficiencies and features are analysed. Patients, physicians, hospital managers and healthcare policy-makers all define 'healthcare quality' from their perspectives though they may judge quality in the same way. A way out of such a dilemma in defining quality would be based on 'radical constructivism'. Deducing from radical constructivism quality can be defined as a 'construct' which would incorporate quality dimensions important to various stakeholders. In turn, the quality management programmes can operationalize the construct much more effectively and satisfy the needs of different stakeholders.

3

Quality Assurance in Healthcare

In Chapter 2, it was discussed and agreed upon that 'quality of care' be best defined in terms of technical standards and specifications as well as service components in order to meet patient's satisfaction. We also examined that no single definition of healthcare service quality applies to all situations and that 'quality as a construct' is a more comprehensive definition. Such an approach would ensure and meet the expectations of multiple stakeholders. It would also fulfil the criteria that the quality of care should achieve the most favourable balance of benefits and risks. This means benefits should be maximized without correspondingly increasing risks. In case of community and public health, interventions should be as per standards and affordable, and impact mortality, morbidity, disability and malnutrition. Quality of care should be defined in light of both technical standards and patients' expectations. Focus on client/patient, systems and processes, measurement and teamwork forms the core of any assurance programme. Figure 3.1 depicts the simplest way to view Quality Assurance (QA) mechanism. The QA triangle illustrates the core functions of quality management, namely 'defining quality', 'measuring quality against set standards' and 'improving quality' when gap arises. QA programmes can achieve synergy when all the three activities are implemented in a coordinated fashion. This chapter discusses the QA in healthcare and critically evaluates its effectiveness. The last section of the chapter highlights the limitations of QA and makes a case for implementation of Total Quality Management (TQM) in healthcare organizations.

Figure 3.1
Quality Assurance Triangle

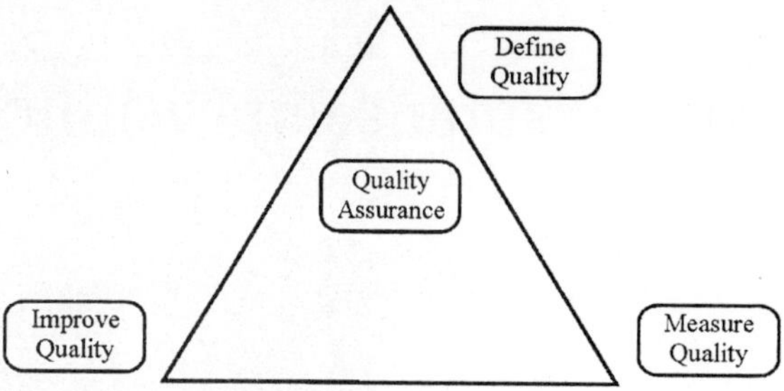

Source: The Quality Assurance Project (QAP) funded by the US Agency for International Development (USAID) under Contract Number GPH-C-00-02-00004-00, available at http://www.qaproject.org/methods/resqamodel.html

Quality Assurance in Healthcare

Fundamental approaches to managing quality can be broadly viewed under two categories: Quality Assurance (QA) and Total Quality Management (TQM) also referred to as Continuous Quality Improvement (CQI). QA is based essentially on standards agreed by experts in the field or statutory in nature. It will focus on defining the components of a service (staff qualifications, size of buildings, access to journals, etc.) and the processes to be followed (committees to be set up, data to be collected, protocols to be prepared). Regular external inspections are performed to ensure that standards are being followed. The assumption is that if the standards are being followed, and if they were correctly defined then through the process of review, a high quality of service will follow. Such QA mechanisms include different forms of external review such as accreditation, inspection, regulation, audit or external peer review (Potter et al., 1994; Walshe et al., 2001). BS 5750 and USA's JCAHO accreditation systems are examples of QA approaches. NHS in England uses the external review very widely including medical training inspection, ISO 9000 quality management, external quality awards (such as 'Investors in People' and the Chartermark) and a number of accreditation schemes for different types of healthcare organizations (Thomson and Hodgson, 1997; Walshe et al., 2001). 'ExPeRT', a European Union project on external peer review techniques, researched the scope, mechanisms and use of external quality mechanisms in the improvement of healthcare (Shaw, 2000). National Accreditation Board of India (NABH) in India will be discussed in Chapter 5 in detail. It indicates that patients, public at large and many corporate bodies are promoting external quality mechanisms at the national level. Table 3.1 shows the various groups of stakeholders and their concerns in terms of quality of healthcare.

Table 3.1

Corporate Stakeholders and their Concerns in External Quality Mechanisms

Stakeholder	*Primary Concern*
Government	Health policy
Statutory bodies	Registration
Healthcare providers	Management
Insurers	Funding
Membership societies	Quality improvement
Professions	Education, self-regulation
Consumer organizations	Public information

Source: Shaw, 2000, p. 171.

'ExPeRT' categorized the *organizational standards* into four groups based on purpose of the models developed: *professional performance* (e.g., visitation, *visitatie* in Dutch; medical audits in hospitals); *health service delivery* (e.g., accreditation schemes); *management system* (e.g., EFQM) and quality systems (e.g., ISO). QA programmes were introduced in hospitals in the mid-1970s as part of the accreditation requirements in both the US and Canada. Initially, they were required only for medical staff but were gradually extended to all areas. By the mid-1980s, hospitals were required to have comprehensive and coordinated, hospital-wide quality programmes (Short and Rahim, 1995). In general, QA programmes are professional dominated, except ISO that was not initially intended for healthcare organizations. The following section discusses the most important QA mechanisms, namely, accreditation, audit methods and ISO.

Accreditation of Healthcare Organizations

Accreditation is one of the most popular external mechanisms of QA in healthcare. In general, accreditation is a process in which an entity, separate and distinct from the healthcare organization, usually non-governmental, assesses the healthcare organization to determine if it meets a set of standards and requirements designed to improve the quality of care. Accreditation is usually voluntary and standards are regarded as optimal and achievable. On the part of the healthcare organization, accreditation provides a visible commitment by an organization to improve the quality of patient care, to ensure a safe environment and to reduce risks to patients and staff. As one examines the accreditation of healthcare organizations, a wide variety of methods exist across the nations and Table 3.2 highlights the meanings as used by different groups.

Table 3.2

Meanings of 'Accreditation' as Used by Different Professional Groups and Constituencies

Group	*Intended Meaning*	*Since (Century/Year)*
Professional bodies	Recognition of speciality training	19th Century
Consortia of clinicians and managers	Recognition of service delivery	c1920
International Organization for standardization	Recognition of agency competent to certificate healthcare providers	1946

Source: Shaw, 2000, p. 171.

Hurst (1997) discussed the characteristics of healthcare accreditation schemes in the UK and concluded that the King's Fund Organizational Audit is perhaps the most established audit method. He identified 16 approaches from various sources that are being used for healthcare in the UK such as British Standard ISO 9000, Charter Mark, Health Advisory Service for Elderly Psychiatric Care, King's Fund Organizational Audit, Professional education bodies such as the Medical Royal Colleges and the National Boards for Nursing, Trent Small-Hospital Accreditation Schemes, etc.

At the international level, Joint Commission on Accreditation of Healthcare Organizations (JCAHO) along with its Joint Commission International (JCI) has become an important accrediting agency for hospitals. Joint Commission on Accreditation of Healthcare Organizations is one of the most credible accrediting organizations and has been a major force in setting QA standards in healthcare organizations in the US. The standards were developed in the USA from 1917 as a mechanism for recognition of training posts in surgery. That model was the beginning of JCAHO; it was exported via Canada to Australia in the 1970s and arrived in Europe in the 1980s. It is most evident in the UK, Spain, Portugal, The Netherlands and Finland and, by statute, in Italy and France. It is being developed in Switzerland (by the Swiss Society for Quality in Health Care) and Germany (jointly by the Medical Chamber and insurance companies) (Shaw, 2000). The mission of JCAHO is to continuously improve the safety and quality of care provided to the public through the provision of healthcare accreditation and related services that support performance improvement in healthcare organizations.

Initially, JCAHO emphasized establishing proper environment for providing high-quality care, rather than determining if high-quality care was actually being provided. Later, the focus shifted from structure to process. Around 1980s, the standards did not indicate how potential problems were to be identified or addressed. But, the hospital QA personnel were asked to identify problems, set goals, focus on errors in the process of care and demonstrate that they had met their own goals. Therefore, many hospitals focused on issues that could be easily resolved. Also, many hospitals primarily structured and focused their QA activities primarily toward compliance with JCAHO survey/guidelines. Since the society has delegated the establishment of quality standards to medical profession, JCAHO's approach is supposed to reflect the values of society (DesHarnais and McLaughlin, 1999).

In response to the growing interest in accreditation and quality improvement worldwide, the Joint Commission launched its international accreditation programme in 1999. Joint Commission International (JCI) accreditation standards are based on international consensus standards and set uniform, achievable expectations for structures, processes and outcomes for hospitals.

The accreditation process is designed to accommodate specific legal, religious and cultural factors within a country. International Standards for Hospitals in Europe, South America, Asia and the Middle East; International Standards for Clinical Laboratories, Care Continuum, Medical Transport Organization, Disease or Condition-Specific Standards and recently for Ambulatory Care are available. Joint Commission International helps to improve the quality of patient care in many nations through international consultation, accreditation, publications and education. Joint Commission International requirements focus on staff management (job description, appointment process and crediting competence) and care activities management (admission, discharge and transfer, delivery of high-risk services).

A number of limitations of accreditation are identified from literature and are summarized below:

- Accreditation is primarily medical profession based in its approach. Medical professionals have retained a high level of autonomy to determine the working conditions and terms of payment. This in turn has helped turn medical decision-making into a 'black box', which has become relatively immune to outside examination (ibid.).
- Joint Commission on Accreditation of Healthcare Organization review would pay particular attention to effects and control such as adverse events and respect of patient's rights. But market may be not a primary concern for healthcare managers as marketing and financial aspects are rather less developed (ibid.).
- Eggli and Halfon (2003) have noted that data-driven improvement activities are emphasized in JCAHO type of accreditation, but evaluation requirements are relatively weak and that benchmarking embedded in other models such as EFQM is lacking. Even standards do not apply to specifically clinical practices probably owing to a lack of confidence in the validity of the quality indicators.
- Based on works on accreditation in healthcare, Scrivens has expressed the following concerns about accreditation schemes in general: The coverage of accreditation schemes is uneven; there is no consensus about standard and good

practice; there is conflict between accreditation schemes; accreditation boards work in different ways; the differences between accreditation reports and grades make the task of evaluating the nature and purpose of accreditation more difficult (Scrivens, 1995, cited in Hurst, 1997).

Audit Methods

Majority of the healthcare organizations use some form of audit methods to ensure quality of healthcare services. Audits based on clinical indicators such as hospital infection rates, nosocomial infections, surgical site infections, etc. are most common. NHS of the UK is one of the healthcare systems in the world which uses audit methods extensively. In the UK, quality initiatives and reforms themselves have taken the form of Medical Audit, Clinical Audit, Clinical Governance, The Patient's Charter, Re-engineering and Total Quality Management (Newman, 1997; Thomson and Hodgson, 1997; Donaldson and Gray, 1998; Leatherman and Sutherland, 1998; Sutherland and Dawson, 1998; Collins et al., 2000; Zairi and Jarrar, 2001; Ritchie, 2002).

Medical audit is used as the main professional method for assessing the quality of clinical practice. Medical audit is defined as "a systematic quantified comparison against explicit standards in current medical practice in order to improve the quality of care to patients" (Shaw, 1990 cited in Thomson and Hodgson, 1997). Royal Colleges and Faculties supported widely the medical audit and defined it as "the systematic, critical analysis of the quality of medical care including procedures used for diagnosis and treatment, the use of resources and the resulting outcome and quality of life for the patient". Though the definition emphasizes some key points, it fails to ensure audit as a change management process and does not mention the importance of explicit standards. In the NHS, the uni-disciplinary medical audit moved toward 'clinical audit' which involves the entire healthcare team.

Thomson and Hodgson (1997) have described the following important audit methods for medical services:

- *Critical incident discussion* might involve clinical peers discussing unexpected complications or deaths to identify problems and potential changes in practice. This usually concentrates on individual cases and less amenable around audit cycle (Figure 3.2).

- *Case note review audit* concentrates on the quality of the medical record, which could be improved. There was a lot of initial enthusiasm in the UK for this method but it is known to become repetitive and tedious.
- *Critical event monitoring* measures the rates of critical events, such as wound infection or mortality rates. Audit cycle can be more effectively used with this (Figure 3.2).

Figure 3.2
The Audit Cycle

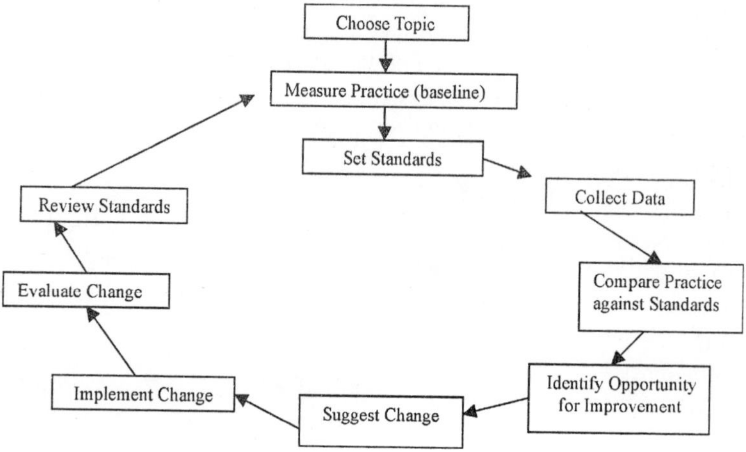

Source: Thomson and Hodgson, 1997, p. 141.

- *Other routine monitoring* can include monitoring of positive events or outcomes such as patient satisfaction or change in health status.
- *Criterion-based topic review* is a type of audit in which a set of standards (or protocols or guidelines) is agreed for the management of a specific symptom or diagnostic group and the collected data are reviewed with those standards.

The topic of audit in healthcare in the UK has become both complex and problematic (Brown and Bell, 1998). Drawbacks and problems with audit are summarized thus:

- Audit methods are found to be burdensome in clinical practice and some complain it as repetitive and boring;
- Audit's value is not clear and enormous financial and opportunity costs of routine audit have not been justified.
- Though the potential benefits of audit methods cannot be denied, audit and external review mechanisms are not adequately researched (Thomson and Hodgson, 1997; Walshe et al., 2001). Integration of audit into routine clinical practice and the mechanisms are important issues to be addressed.
- Varieties of audit (medical, clinical, managerial and professional audits) used in NHS in the UK do not traditionally include the patient's perspective. There is a need to bridge the gap between the health quality literature and modern views of quality grounded in patients' views (Brown and Bell, 1998).

As quality management has evolved over the last three to four decades, a number of people have examined the changes and moved toward clinical governance in NHS (Donaldson and Gray, 1998; Leatherman and Sutherland, 1998; Sutherland and Dawson, 1998; Beecham, 1999; Ritchie, 2002). Clinical governance is "a framework through which local organizations are accountable for continuously improving the quality of their services and safeguarding high standards of care by creating an environment in which excellence in clinical care will flourish" (Clinical Governance: Quality in the new NHS; Department of Health, UK, 1998 cited in Beecham, 1999). According to Beecham (1999), for clinical governance to be successful it is suggested that "... all healthcare organizations must have an open culture in which education, research, and sharing of good practice are valued and expected; a commitment to quality that is shared by staff and managers; a tradition of actively working with patients, users, care givers, and the public; the ethos of multidisciplinary teamwork at all levels; and regular board level discussions of all major quality issues". Four principles of the clinical governance are:

- responsibility and accountability,
- comprehensive quality improvement (an evaluation culture),

- risk management (self-assessment of risk and minimizing clinical risk), and
- identification and remedy of poor performance.

It is clear that clinical governance is a major shift from audit to more proactive culture strategy from that of blaming to one of learning. This would be more conducive for ensuring high quality medical care (Houghton and Wall, 2000). Therefore, there is a shift toward the TQM approach rather than assurance mechanisms. The next section examines the ISO certification for hospitals as a QA mechanism and discusses its uses and limitations.

International Standardization Organization (ISO)

This international body works for developing various standards (mostly for products) for bringing uniformity and request their member countries to ratify the standards and implement them. Most of the countries including India are members of the ISO. It enlists the technical specifications to be met by a product before the same is certified. The ISO developed standards for quality systems (ISO 9000 series) which have been used to assess specific aspects of health services, particularly in Germany and Switzerland. Because the standards relate to administrative procedures rather than clinical results, ISO has been used more often in mechanical departments such as laboratories (EN 45001), radiology and transport, but it is being increasingly applied to whole hospitals and clinics recently (Shaw, 2000). Over the past few years, many hospitals in India have started/achieved accreditation under the ISO. Gyani and Mittal (2001) have given a detailed outline for the application of ISO 9001: 2000 to the health sector particularly to hospitals. In general, ISO focuses on documentation of management systems and the development of ISO is driven by existing users, however, most of them are not related to healthcare.

There are three kinds of certificates available under ISO 9000 scheme, namely, ISO 9001, ISO 9002 and ISO 9003. These certificates are not awarded to a product but to a system. The hospital, too, is a system and therefore, it can get ISO certification. ISO 9004 is not a standard but is a set of guidelines which help toward working for the establishment of a quality system. Some of the reputed hospitals are providing innovative services by designing processes. But, normally, majority of the hospitals do not do so and they act as providers of the existing services and, therefore, ISO-9002 is the most suitable certification for a hospital. Table 3.3 below gives the details of various ISO schemes available:

Table 3.3

The ISO 9000 Series

Standard	*Focus*
Original Standard (ISO 9000)	
ISO 9000	Quality management and assurance standards for selection and use.
ISO 9001	Quality systems model for quality assurance in organizations whose processes include design, development, production, installation and servicing.
ISO 9002	Quality systems model for quality assurance in organizations whose processes include production and installation, but not design and development.
ISO 9003	Quality systems model for quality assurance in organizations whose processes use final inspection and testing to meet product and service quality requirements.
ISO 9004	Quality management and quality system guidelines.
Revised Standards (ISO 9000)	
ISO 9000: 2000	Quality management system fundamentals and vocabulary – defines terminology and standards.
ISO 9001: 2000	Quality management systems requirements – used to assess compliance with requirements (consolidates the former ISO 9001/9002/9003 into a single document).
ISO 9004: 2000	Quality management systems guidelines for performance improvement – offers guidance for continual management system improvement.

Source: Magd and Curry, 2003, p. 245.

ISO 9000 depends mainly upon policies and documentation as an evidence of QA activity. An accrediting team assesses the applicant and further assessment visits occur at intervals. The ISO 9000 registration and kite mark can be withdrawn if the standards are not met. Though the value of ISO 9000 lies in its enforcement of a systematic organization-wide approach, there are problems with requirements of documentation and systems development. Furthermore, ISO 9000 in itself may not change attitudes within an organization. A number of researchers have identified the limitations of ISO standards and argue for a more comprehensive TQM model to achieve excellence in quality. They are:

- The ISO 9000 organizations focus on standards and understanding processes for technical requirements and achieve certification. But, non-technical aspects like people and leadership style are not focused (Low, 1998). Work by Priebe (2000) identified that the reliance on external standards such as ISO 9000 allows organizations to shift responsibility for quality issues to external authorities and creates a 'compliance mentality' throughout the organization. Further, Priebe (2000) concluded that a philosophy change and a comprehensive exercise involving all levels of the healthcare system, and not just a mere technique to be applied through external pressure would be more valuable.
- Magd and Curry (2003) through an extensive literature survey on ISO and TQM have concluded that no longer quality is merely a concept of meeting customer's expectations but of exceeding them. Quality is not just about 'what is offered' (product or service) but also about 'how it is offered'. ISO 9000 concentrates on processes and attaches great importance to the management of quality in suppliers and in all the manufacturing processes including the design and the specifications that the products and services should achieve. In reality, understanding of customer is important in product or service design (Lozano, 1997).
- Eggli and Halfon (2003) have noted that the main objective of ISO is to put the client's mind at rest. Most ISO requirements focus on activities of management including description and measure of processes, noted quality standards, prevention and correction of errors, product traceability and document control, and on effects which are monitored in terms of customer satisfaction. The ISO is more prevalent in European countries wherein health systems depend a lot on government regulation and professional norms as drivers for improving quality than the US wherein the system is more customer and market driven.
- The ISO provides a common basis for assuring buyers that specific practices are in conformance with the provider's

stated quality systems and does not address what should be improved in order to gain a company's competitive position (Zhu and Scheuermann, 1999).

- If an organization's goal is to maintain ISO certification then the key is to minimize non-conformance by controlling culture (or restricting). However, if flexibility and innovations are the goals then the organization is better guided by TQM principles (Hind, 1996).
- Based on an empirical research, Tarì (2005) found that the human issues and continuous improvement activities are least implemented components in ISO firms in Spain. Incidentally, those issues are only briefly dealt with by the ISO 9000 norm. In addition, social concerns and quality planning were found to be the weakest areas in those firms. The author concluded that if the final objective was to maintain the ISO 9000 certificate they would stay at the basic TQM level. In order to improve competitiveness, the logical next step could be to use a TQM model such as EFQM to define improvement activities.

Limitations of Quality Assurance

Quality management of hospitals and healthcare organizations are based on QA methods in general. The above literature review discussed accreditation, audit methods and ISO certification. Though quality assurance is found useful by the organizations, it has the following major limitations:

- *QA is driven by standards and stresses conformance to standards.* In general, QA involves a group of in-house professionals checking for compliance and identifying problem areas based on sporadic visits and not necessarily on a continuous basis. QA's ability to ensure continuous quality improvement or motivating staff to become quality conscious (except in the short term to achieve accreditation) is less certain. In fact, in the US and Australia there has been a major shift of orientation toward 'clinical indicators' because quality assurance and accreditation have led to a plateau of standards that have not kept pace with public expectations (Potter et al., 1994).

- QA assumes that the *agency of quality assurance knows the best* and should dictate what good quality means. Universal 'one size fits all' review approaches, in which the same methodology is used for all reviewed organizations regardless of their nature or context, seem to be at best wasteful of resources and perhaps even positively harmful (Walshe et al., 2001).
- It means *preparing for an announced visit* from an accrediting agency (often a time-consuming task) by staging a show to reflect good quality assurance. The process itself could be inherently inspectorial, summative and judgemental, at least from the organization's point of view. Inspection overload leads to a degree of confusion, fatigue and cynicism about the process within the reviewed organization, and it may detract from rather than adding to the quality of care (ibid.).
- Most QA activities are *driven by episodic measurement*. It provides a fire-fighting kind of mechanism rather than focus on process generating episodes and process management throughout the organization. External review rarely generates new knowledge about an organization, but rather it makes explicit or known to others information that already exists (ibid.).
- In general, *QA utilizes judgemental and subjective evaluations*; it does not use numbers or data on facts. The study by Washe et al. (2001) indicated that external reviews can be costly, and the review process is relatively subjective and open to bias.
- It is pointed out that once the certification is over, there is a *general tendency for organizations to revert back to original ways* of carrying on with business. Collingwood (1996) comments that "... in their search for the elusive perfect system of quality assurance (QA), managers everywhere have been diverted from the goals of their organization. Their desire to demonstrate with a flag, kite, or some other accreditation emblem, that they have a 'quality' organization, has increased the organizational bureaucracy and taken attention from their real purpose – the attainment of organizational goal". A hospital's logo with a quality

standard met does nothing more than the fact that time and money has been spent on enhancing the existing bureaucracy and developing a management system.

- Even when external review is intended to be developmental and supportive, those at the sharp end often *perceive it as summative and potentially punitive*. The Walshe et al. (2001) concluded that "... external reviews rarely generated wholly new knowledge, were more confirmatory than revelatory, and did not usually lead to major changes in policy, strategy or practice".

Improving Quality Systems in Healthcare

Owing to the limitations and problems associated with QA, hospital managers are trying to use innovative methods and learn from TQM experiences of other industries. Short and Rahim (1995) have summarized the differences between QA and TQM as given in Table 3.4. It clearly indicates that TQM approach can help organizations overcome a number of limitations and problems associated with traditional QA approaches.

Table 3.4

Comparison of Total Quality Management and Quality Assurance in Healthcare

Aspect	*TQM Approach*	*QA Approach*
General Orientation	Assumption of need to improve precedes measurement	Monitoring and measurement performed to identify needs for improvement
	Proactive	Reactive
	Variation prevention	Variation detection
	Customer	Provider
Commitment	Heavily stressed and of paramount importance, evident at all levels with senior level leadership	Not overly stressed as a critical component
Focus	Total organization	Clinical areas
	Improving average performance	Improving outlier performance

Cont'd...

Cont'd...

	Common cause	Special cause
	Systems and processes	Provider or practitioner
	Input, process and output element of product or service delivery	Structure, process, outcome elements of critical functions with added dimensions of appropriateness, risk minimization and clinical performance
Structure	Uses existing structure with cross-functional team	Superimposes separate QA structure
Requirements and specifications	Customer defined	Provider defined
Use of standards and norms	The standard is the starting point	The standard is the goal
Quality costs	Emphasized	Not emphasized
Mass inspection	Promotes elimination of mass inspection	Promotes broad based inspections and adequate sampling
Use of statistical methods	Sophisticated	Rudimentary

Source: Short and Rahim, 1995, p. 262.

Harteloh (2003) has explored the use of a socio-technical approach characterized as bottom up, incremental, information technology facilitated and indicator driven (in the lines of TQM) in order to construct quality systems as an alternative to the traditional ISO-oriented approach. In healthcare, he strongly argues that quality indicators (e.g., unexpected readmissions, avoidable mortality, unscheduled return to OR or ICU, patient satisfaction, costs, quality of life, etc.) conceptualize the theory of meaning and therefore constructing a system by developing relevant indicators is important for quality. From a socio-technical point of view, a quality system is an association, a network of humans and artefacts. The differences in the approaches of ISO and socio-technical system are presented in Table 3.5.

The above discussion highlights the importance of quality management based on a socio-technical approach of TQM rather than the QA approach. As organizations gained experience and fine tuned their quality management methods in general, importance of continuous improvement based on measurement and analysis of quality data, organizational learning and cost effective approaches became clear.

Table 3.5

Constructing Quality Systems in Healthcare

	Formal (ISO) Oriented Approach	*Socio-technical Approach*
Theoretical basis	General systems theory	A theory of meaning
Purpose	External accountability by standardization and certification	Stimulating and facilitating internal reflexivity of the organization
Construction (by)	Describing elements and their formal relationships (External) blueprint Organizational diagnosis	Dialogue
	Stepwise strategy, according to a plan or blueprint	Needs of healthcare workers and patients Change in relationships between actors. Incremental strategy, according to politics or social dynamics
Implementation	Top down Project, scheduled in time Standard driven Facilitated by education and training Guided by external advise	Bottom up Continuous growth Indicator driven IT facilitated learning innovation Guided by qualitative research and participation
Meaning	Quality as a (static) property Formal interpretation (procedure)	Quality as (dynamic) capacity Focus on information Social interpretation (quality circle)

Source: Harteloh, 2003, p. 394.

Thornber (cited in Short and Rahim, 1995) defined TQM as a method of leadership and management which:

- defines quality in terms of customer perceptions of both the content and delivery of the service;

- analyses systems for errors and variation rather than blaming people;
- develops long-term partnerships with external and internal suppliers;
- uses accurate data to analyse processes and measure system improvement;
- involves the staff who work in the system analysis and improvement;
- sets up effective collaborative meetings as the basis of teamwork;
- trains supervisors and managers in leading the on-going improvement process;
- engages staff in setting targets and ensures that results are fed back;
- highlights the need for senior executives to plan strategically; and
- achieves long-term improvement through small incremental steps.

The next chapter describes the works of quality gurus and later examines the emergence of TQM in healthcare.

Summary

QA mechanisms are extensively used in healthcare service for quality management. The chapter closely examined accreditation, medical audits and ISO approaches of QA. Their applications and limitations were critically assessed. In the context of liberalization, globalization, competition and consumer awareness, the healthcare organizations can no longer ignore the quality of services they provide. Often, healthcare organizations are seen to move from inspection-oriented quality improvement system to one that orients itself to a systematic transformation of organizational culture through a comprehensive plan involving customer focus, key-process monitoring, data-driven tools, and techniques and team empowerment.

4

Total Quality Management in Healthcare

In the light of increasing internationalization, liberalization, deregulation and competition, organizations striving for competitive success have searched for and adopted new management forms and philosophies. A prime example of this has been the widespread adoption and implementation of quality programmes. In the early 1970s, Quality was the key when the American industry was struggling hard to counter the success of Japanese consumer products such as personal computers and consumer electronics. By mid-1980s, the usefulness and success of TQM had become increasingly obvious and well documented in the manufacturing industry. In the following sections, works of the major contributors to TQM are presented. Later, emergence of TQM in healthcare, important elements and applications are discussed in depth.

Emergence of Total Quality Management Concepts

The fundamentals of TQM are based on scientific management movement began at the turn of the century. The idea of 'management based on facts' gained ground. It became well accepted that there exists 'one correct method of work' and that ensuring that all personnel executed that method would lead to quality. Gradually, human relation perspective gained importance in achieving total quality. Most histories of TQM have credited statistics part to the pioneering works of Walter Shewart at Bell Laboratories. His best-known contributions are the control chart and the Plan, Do, Check, Act (PDCA) cycle. Pioneers of TQM such as Deming, Juran, Crosby and Ishikawa have come to be known as 'quality gurus' (McGlaughlin and Kaluzny, 1999; Haigh, 2000; Krüger, 2001; Logothetis, 2003; Mohanty and Lakhe, 2006). The US and Japanese *quality gurus* have contributed a number of important ideas to today's understanding TQM. Berwick (1991, p. 420) emphasizes that the TQM approach with its multidisciplinary emphasis is suited to clinical care as it is "a network of deep interdependencies involving other professionals, non-professional staff, information systems, policies and procedures, physical systems, and other influences on their own work and the patients they serve. Sometimes physicians indeed act alone, but usually not".

The main thesis of Deming is: by improving quality it is possible to increase productivity which results in the improved competitiveness of a business enterprise. In order to achieve this aim, Deming (1950s onwards) developed an approach with the now famous 14-point programme (e.g., create constancy of purpose for continual improvement of product and service; cease dependence on inspection to achieve quality; end practice of awarding business on price tag alone; etc.). He further noted that quality does not come from inspection, but from improvement of the company's work processes. He iterated that it is important to 'build good quality in' rather than 'inspect bad quality out'. Deming's programme stresses training and instilling a need for TQM culture among the workforce. Krüger (2001) has pointed out that statistical methods remain the heart of Deming's ideas though there was an attempt to recognize a holistic quality management system. However, Deming does not consider certain aspects of today's TQM approach, such as positively motivating the individual employee to dedicate himself to quality work.

Juran's (1950s) quality control approach definitely has the managerial aspect, his main contribution being "quality control must be conducted as an integral part of the management function" (Krüger, 2001). This is evident from the Juran's recommendations for the management to establish Quality Council as a central coordinating team to enhance quality activities of the organization. Further, quality policy and quality goals should be set and that the management should ensure resources and mechanisms to achieve those goals. Juran thus broadened the understanding of quality at that time by making it an integral part of management function.

Feigenbaum's approach to TQM includes elements such as management of quality, the system for total quality, management strategies and quality, engineering technology and quality, statistical technology and the application of total quality in the enterprise. He contributed two new aspects to quality discussion, first, quality is the responsibility of everybody in the company ranging from top management to the unskilled worker. According to him, long-term business success is possible with total participation of all employees and the total integration of all the company's technical and human resources. Second, he was the first to recognize that costs of non-quality have to be categorized and measured for better management. They are costs of control and costs of failure of control. Costs of control can be measured in two principle areas, namely, prevention costs (e.g., quality training of employees) and appraisal costs (e.g., quality audit costs). Costs of failure can also be measured in two areas: internal failure costs (e.g., scrap) and external failure costs (e.g., customer complaints, reworked material). This means that postproduction inspection syndrome does not make any allowance for the prevention of defective parts during the production process itself. However, his highly structured approach to total quality hardly covers the question of motivation and commitment of the individual employee to quality.

Crosby's works in the 1980s emphasized *zero defects and do it right the first time* as the only standards of performance, any other *acceptable quality levels (AQL)* are not good enough. His famous concept "Quality is free. It is not a gift, but it is free. What costs money is the unquality things – all the actions that involve not doing jobs right the first time" is very popular in the TQM literature. He makes it clear that quality has only to be defined as 'conformance to requirements'. He further says that quality is the responsibility of every employee in the company and not of the quality department which has no control or immediate access to. Crosby offers his 'quality vaccine' for business enterprises to prevent the problem of non-conformance. He recommends applying his four absolutes of quality management: (i) do it right the first time; (ii) the system of quality is prevention; (iii) the performance standard is 'zero defects'; and (iv) the measurement of quality is the price of non-conformance. Crosby, however, does not make any reference to the actual quality tools and techniques required to realizing his concept.

The work of Ishikawa influenced the Japanese understanding of quality. He is known for the four aspects of TQM: quality circles, the question of continuous training, the quality tool *Ishikawa diagram (cause & effect diagram)* and the quality chain. In his definition of TQM, he emphasizes a clear customer orientation (internal and external), involvement of all departments and everyone in the company, and top management to lead by example. He further claims that TQM begins with education and ends with education. One can agree to the fact that Ishikawa has contributed and formed a number of important ideas of today's understanding of TQM.

Ishikawa and other Japanese engineers refined the application of the foundations of CQI and added the following features (McLaughlin and Kaluzny, 1999):

1. Total participation by all members of an organization (quality must be company-wide).
2. Identifying the next step of a process as its customer just as the preceding step is its supplier.
3. The necessity of communicating with both the customer and the supplier (promoting feedback and creating channels of communication throughout the system).
4. A participative team emphasis, starting with quality circles.
5. An emphasis on education and training.
6. Quality audits, e.g., the Deming Prize.
7. Rigorous use of statistics.
8. 'Just in time' processes.

As the TQM approaches are revised and adapted, increasing innovation and experimentation have evolved. In healthcare, too, such attempts are very common as hospitals try their best to apply TQM. Table 4.1 presents a comparison of quality gurus, namely, Crosby, Deming and Juran on various dimensions of definition, approach, structure and other factors. The views can help guide any organization setting upon the path which leads to becoming a quality organization.

Table 4.1

Quality Gurus Compared

	Crosby	*Deming*	*Juran*
Definition of quality	Conformance to requirements	A predictable of uniformity and dependability at low cost and suited to the market	Fitness for use
Degree of senior management responsibility	Responsible for quality	Responsible for 94% of quality problems	Less than 20% of quality problems are due to workers
Performance standard/ motivation	Zero defects	Quality has many 'scales'; use statistics to measure performance in all areas; critical of zero defects	Avoid campaigns to 'do perfect work'
General approach	Prevention, not inspection	Reduce variability by continuous improvement; cease mass inspection	General management approach to quality, especially 'human' elements
Structure	14 steps to quality improvement	14 points for management	10 steps to quality improvement
Statistical process control (SPC)	Rejects statistically acceptable levels of quality	Statistical methods of quality control must be used	Recommends SPC but warns that it can lead to 'tool-driven' approach
Improvement basis	A 'process', not a programme; improvement goals	Continuous to reduce variation; eliminate goals without methods	Project-by-project team approach; set goals
Teamwork	Quality improvement teams; quality councils	Employee participation in decision-making; break down barriers between departments	Team and quality circle approach

Cont'd...

Cont'd...

Coast of quality	Cost of non-conformation; quality is free	No optimum, continuous improvement	Quality is not free, there is an optimum
Purchasing and goods received	State requirements; supplier is extension of business; most faults due to purchasers themselves	Inspection too late; allows defects to enter system through AQLs; statistical evidence and control charts required	Problems are complex; carry out formal surveys
Vendor rating	Yes and buyers; quality audits useless	No, critical of most systems	Yes, but help supplier improve
Single sourcing of supply		Yes	No, can neglect to sharpen competitive edge

Source: Adapted from Haigh, 2000, p. S591.

Tracing Total Quality Management in Healthcare

Quality is a central issue in healthcare organizations and will continue to be so. In the 1960s and 1970s, healthcare was still considered a cottage industry. That is, "healthcare was delivered by individual professionals who practised a craft or art, who learned by apprenticeship, worked independently in a decentralized system, tailored their craft to each individual situation using processes which were not recorded nor explicitly engineered, and were personally accountable for the performance and financial outcomes" (McLaughlin and Kaluzny, 1999, p. 11). During 1980s and 1990s, a decided change was seen – *industrialization of healthcare* (in India, this phenomenon is seen from mid-1990s). These changes have affected almost all aspects of healthcare delivery: the way risks are allocated, how care is organized, and how professionals are motivated and incentivized.

Further, it can be seen that *corporatization of healthcare* has been redefined and will continue to redefine how quality is managed. The view that healthcare is an *economic good* (with more spending on health by countries) has influenced how healthcare organizations are professionally managed comparable to organizations in the industrial sector. For instance, 'marketing' functions not so stressed in hospitals are very much a part now. The use of titles such as President, Chief Executive Officer or Chief of Operations rather than Administrator is becoming more prevalent. In the area of quality management, nomenclature and perspective known as TQM is being applied in the healthcare. Though the components of TQM approach are not antithetical to the way that quality has been defined and managed within healthcare services, there are some important differences from that of industries (McLaughlin and Kaluzny, 1999).

Quality approaches and organization developments go hand in hand. Using the Victor and Boynton (1998) model for arriving at an appropriate path for organizational development and improvement, McLaughlin and Kaluzny (1999) provided insights into different quality approaches that are suitable to various stages of healthcare processes and product lines. The stages of development of services/products are: craft (invention) stage, mass production, process enhancement, mass customization and co-configuration (Figure 4.1).

Figure 4.1

Revised Boynton and Victor Model for Healthcare

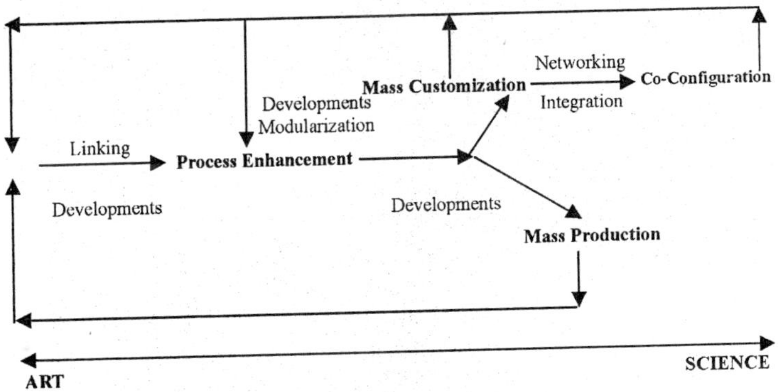

Source: McLaughlin and Kaluzny, 1999, p. 15.

1. While practising any craft, individuals improve with experience. The tacit knowledge developed over a period of time is used to enhance individual reputation and group reputation (i.e., doctor as an individual and 'doctors

community'). Here, strict practice guidelines are useful for maintaining high standards.

2. Once the production of products (to lesser extent services) is mastered, mass production (e.g., assembly line) is achieved. Mass production requires the discipline that produces conformance quality in high volume at low cost.
3. Production processes once very well understood could lead to process enhancement. It requires that processes be analysed and modified to develop a best practice method approach using worker feedback and process-owning teams within the organization.
4. With process enhancements and customer knowledge, mass customization of products becomes possible. Mass customization requires that the organization takes that best practice, modularizes and supports it independently and then uses those modules to build efficient, low-cost processes that are responsive to individual customer wants and needs.
5. The highest level of process development would be that of co-configuration which involves continuous adaptation to customer intelligence, changing the product to match changing customer needs and wants.

Healthcare is a complex and multi-product environment; hence the developments are not linear. Various types of care can be found at each of five stages, depending on the state of technology and the strategy of the delivery unit. The revolution in healthcare organizations is driven not only by economics, but also by the type of knowledge work that is being done. As scientific information about a healthcare process accumulates, it shifts from the craft to the process enhancement stage. After the process is codified and developed further, it may shift into the mass production mode if the approach is sufficiently cut and dried, the volume is high, and the patients accept this impersonal mode of delivery, e.g., Diagnostic-Related Group (DRG) systems offer almost 500 categories; these rather loose product categories provided the basis for managed care and disease management in the US. This allowed the healthcare providers for the first time to collect and compare outcomes and costs across organizations and processes for many purposes including process enhancement. In fact, the focus of healthcare quality has been process enhancement; the processes can be administrative and/or clinical. Such process enhancement methods in the current healthcare scenario are clinical quality improvement, evidence-based medicine, outcome management and disease management. They rely on clinical epidemiology and joint organizational and professional learning.

Mass customization pathway is best suited for the production of satisfied healthcare customers at low or reasonable costs. At this stage, the organization develops a series of modular approaches to prevention and care, highly articulated and well supported by information technology. They can be deployed efficiently in a variety of places and configurations to respond to customer needs. *Clinical pathways* represent one example of modularization. They represent *best practice* as known to the organization and are applied by a 'configuror' (health professional) to meet the needs of the individual patient. One best example is cataract surgeries which are carried out very effectively at low costs in hospitals (and eye camps in India). This requires an integrated information system, full information about the patient's background, medical history and status. Also, synchronization of the implementation of the service modules to be delivered becomes essential. In a sense, mass customization represents a process that simulates craft, but is highly science-based, coordinated, integrated with other process flows and efficient. The most futuristic stage of this model is 'co-configuration' – a system in which customer is linked into the network and customer intelligence is accessed as readily as the providers. Such modularization would also facilitate quality management more scientifically to minimize variations, improve processes based on data and incorporate TQM principles more effectively in healthcare services.

In the US, the National Demonstration Project in Quality Improvement in Health Care was a collaborative project between industry and healthcare organizations to demonstrate that Continuous Quality Improvement (CQI) could also produce considerable benefit to quality and efficiency of healthcare. Berwick et al. (1990, cited in McLaughlin and Simpson, 1999, pp. 34–35) highlighted 10 key lessons to guide subsequent efforts from the project:

1. Quality improvement tools can work in healthcare.
2. Cross-functional teams are valuable in improving healthcare processes.
3. Data useful for quality improvement abound in healthcare.
4. Quality improvement methods are fun to use.
5. Costs of poor quality are high, and savings are within reach.
6. Involving physicians is difficult.
7. Training needs arise early.
8. Non-clinical processes draw early attention.
9. Healthcare organizations may need broader definitions of quality.
10. In healthcare, as in the manufacturing industry, the success of quality improvement is first of all in the hands of the leaders.

From the US, the TQM implementation has spread to many other parts of the world. As it spread to Europe, there is a difference in both success and pace of quality improvements among countries. Applying organizational theories to understand the differences it was found that the right mix of environmental pressure and the capacity of the organizations to change are required for bringing about significant changes in how healthcare quality is enhanced. In India, quite a lot of interest is generated and hospital managers are trying to implement, at least in some hospitals.

In the case of NHS, UK, following the reforms in an attempt to introduce the philosophies and practice of TQM, the Department of Health provided funding to a number of TQM demonstration sites. The results showed that only two out of the 38 sites had made considerable progress and the majority of the sites had failed to implement a TQM model successfully. It was concluded that TQM could be implemented if a number of problems were addressed. The process of implementation had not received enough investment and investment in training was limited. The degree of commitment leading to a corporate approach varied in most sites (cited in Thomson and Hodgson, 1997, pp. 165–66). Nonetheless, Thomson and Hudgson reiterate that experience suggests that the general approach of TQM is valuable in healthcare.

Elements of Total Quality Management

McLaughlin and Kaluzny (1999, pp. 8–10) have given comprehensive information in TQM (the authors refer to it as CQI). The philosophical, structural and health-care-specific elements capture the distinguishing characteristics of CQI in healthcare setting (see Table 4.2).

General Framework of TQM in Healthcare Organizations

With the success of TQM in the manufacturing sector, services including healthcare initiated a number of programmes on the lines of TQM/CQI. In the US around the mid-1980s, TQM was applied to many healthcare settings. Sixty-nine per cent of the hospitals had begun to implement TQM/CQI by 1993 (Shortell et al., 1995 cited in Castle, 1999, p. 95). McLaughlin and Kaluzny (1999) have identified the early works done by three physicians as most important contributions in this area: Paul Batalden at the Hospital Corporation of America (HCA), Donald Berwick at Harvard Community Health Center and Brent James at Intermountain Health System, all based on the principles outlined by Deming. Deming's basic premise is that management needs to undergo transformation and to manage challenges successfully it is necessary to pursue 'profound knowledge'. Accomplishing transformation requires deliberate learning and incorporation of the knowledge in management. The key elements of the profound knowledge that are highlighted by Deming are:

- appreciation for a system,
- knowledge about variation,
- theory of knowledge, and
- psychology.

According to Deming, knowing the aim of a system, the interrelatedness and interdependency of its components and processes constitute the knowledge of the system. Knowledge of variation is that there is inherent variability of all processes in any product or service production. Knowledge of psychology would include a special focus on understanding the intrinsic motivation that underlies human behaviour. The theory of knowledge specifies

Table 4.2

Distinguishing Characteristics of CQI in Healthcare Setting

Philosophical Elements	*Structural Elements*	*Healthcare-Specific Elements*
1. **Strategic focus:** Having a mission, values and objectives for designing, prioritizing and implementing support for organizational performance.	1. **Process improvement teams:** Forming and empowering teams of employees to deal with existing problems and opportunities.	1. **Epidemiological studies** along with insurance payment and medical records data.
2. **Customer focus:** Focusing on both customer (patient, provider and payer) satisfaction and health outcomes as performance measure.	2. **Seven tools** frequently cited in industrial and health quality literature, flow charts, cause-and-effect diagrams, checksheets, histograms, Pareto charts, control charts and correlational analyses.	2. **Involvement of the medical staff governance process** such as quality assurance, tissue committees, pharmacy and therapeutic committees, and peer review.
3. **Systems view:** Analysis of the whole system, providing a service or influencing an outcome.	3. **Parallel organization:** Development of a separate management structure to set priorities for and monitor CQI strategy and implementation, usually referred to as quality council.	3. Use of risk-adjusted outcome measures.
4. **Data-driven analysis:** Data gathering and using objective data on system operation and systems performance.	4. **Top management commitment:** Leadership to make the process effective and foster its integration into the institutional fabric of the organization.	4. Use of cost-effectiveness analysis.
5. **Implementer involvement:** Involving the owners of all components of the system in seeking a common understanding of its delivery process.	5. **Statistical analysis:** Use of statistics, including statistical process control, to identify and reduce unnecessary variation in processes and practices.	5. Use of quality assurance data and techniques and risk management data.

Cont'd...

Cont'd...

6. **Multiple causation:** Identifying the multiple root causes of a set of system phenomena.	6. **Customer satisfaction measures:** Introduction for market research instruments to monitor customer satisfaction at various levels.	Healthcare managers and professionals can incorporate the traditional healthcare quality initiatives including leadership and values.
7. **Solution identification:** Seeking a set of solutions that enhance overall system performance through simultaneous improvements in a number of normally independent functions.	7. **Benchmarking:** Identification of best practices in related and unrelated settings to emulate as processes or use as performance targets.	
8. **Process optimization:** Optimizing a delivery process to meet customer needs regardless of existing precedents and on implementing the system changes regardless of existing territories and fiefdoms. To quote Dr Edwards Deming: 'Management's job is to optimize the system'.	8. **Redesign processes:** From scratch ensuring that the end product conforms to customer requirements by using techniques of quality function deployment and/or process reengineering.	
9. **Continuing improvement:** Continuing the systems analysis even when a satisfactory solution to the presenting problem is obtained.		
10. **Organizational learning:** Enhancing the capacity of the organization to generate process improvement and foster personal growth.		

Source: McLaughlin and Kaluzny, 1999, pp. 8–10.

that management is prediction (Zabada et al., 1998). Figure 4.2 gives the knowledge linkage required for continual improvement and helps one appreciate the interrelationships. Operationalizing organization transformation based on knowledge and PDCA cycle (Plan, Do, Check and Act) was found very useful. Hospital Corporation of America for instance used PDCA cycle and referred to it as FOCUS-PDCA which provided the health workers a common language and orderly sequence for implementing the cycle of continuous improvement (McLaughlin and Kaluzny, 1999).

Figure 4.2

Knowledge Linkage Required for Continual Improvement

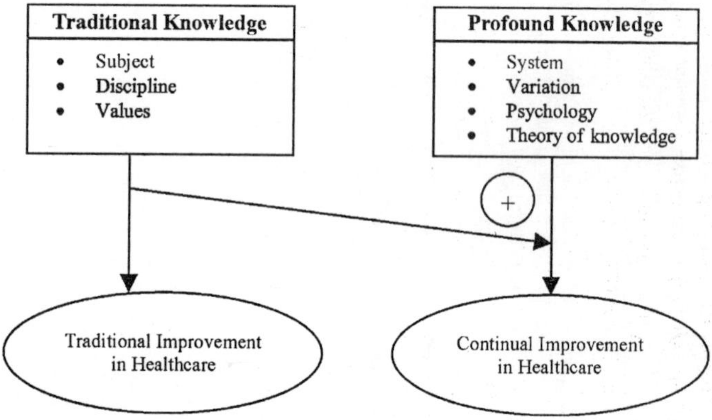

Source: Zabada et al., 1998, p. 64.

In healthcare, the pioneering works of Donabedian not only identified the limitations of industrial model as it ignores or downplays the complexities of the patient – practitioner relationship, professionals' motivation and education/training; quality/cost-trade offs (industrial models treats quality as free), but it also suggested that the professional healthcare model can learn a number of concepts from it. They are: the learning and new appreciation of soundness of healthcare quality traditions, importance of consumers, design of systems and processes for quality, extension of self-monitoring/self-governing tradition of physicians to all in the organization, application of statistical control for monitoring healthcare and greater training/education to all for quality activities.

Donabedian further observed that quality definitions in healthcare generally reflect the values and goals of the current medical care system and of the larger society it is situated in. Donabedian's framework of 'Structure, Process and Outcome' is one of the earliest applied in healthcare quality measurement. He broadened the definition of quality to include not just technical management but also the management of interpersonal relationships, access and continuity of care. The three aspects are:

- *Structure:* the resources available to provide healthcare.
- *Process:* the extent to which professionals perform according to accepted standards.
- *Outcome:* the change in the patient's condition following treatment.

The above approach (Figure 4.3) has advantages and disadvantages. It is easy and relatively simple to monitor structure, for instance, one can do an inventory using a checklist. In fact, external mechanisms for quality assurance agree on minimal structural element standards to ensure an environment. It is obvious that inputs alone will not ensure good outcomes. Process measures take into account professional performance and seem closely related to the outcomes. But outcomes are related to other factors such as patient's condition at the time of treatment, patient compliance and patient age. Provider performance is easy to measure than patient outcomes for many diseases. Process measures can be used to determine whether the professional has performed adequately for specific conditions where there is substantial agreement in what is acceptable care and that the technology is reasonably effective.

Figure 4.3

Donabedian's Model of Quality

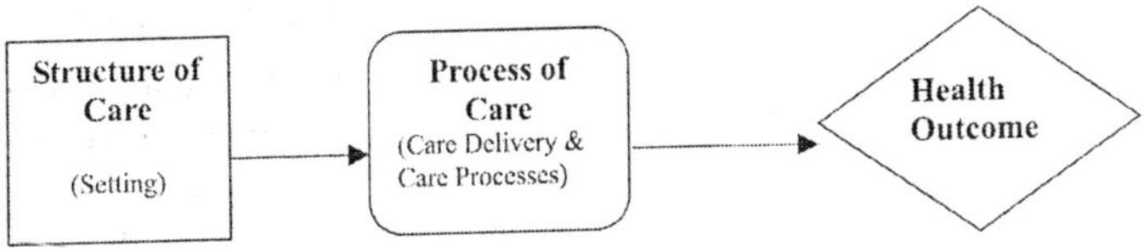

As seen in the above discussion, it is not so straightforward to operationalize the TQM philosophy and integrate continuous improvement into a hospital system which is highly complex. A dialectical approach to understanding TQM can help a researcher realize the applicability of the TQM philosophy. Cunha et al. (2002) provided further insights into TQM as a management of paradoxes. It includes the application of dialectical perspective of *yin-yang* to quality management leading to five principles:

1. less inspection in order to promote product quality,
2. control to promote autonomy,
3. authoritative leadership to promote participation,
4. doubt to promote trust, and
5. routine planning to promote creativity.

The authors further go on to emphasize that "it can be represented by the yin-yang symmetry, which rather than suggesting opposition, conveys an image of continuous action in which the two forces interpenetrate each other in a system of perpetual motion" (Cunha et al., 2002, p. 851). It is strongly felt that the dialectical synthesis would help quality to evolve in the sense of being a theory and praxis, capable of serving its aims as a business tool (e.g., increased efficiency, improvement in addressing client needs) and also as a potential instrument of human development. *Yin* – the intuitive and complex part of quality management can be complimented by the *yang* – rationalism and objectivity.

Advantages of TQM in Hospitals

TQM is a quality-oriented approach that consists of applying a selection of quality management techniques throughout the organization with an aim to increase profitability through customer focus. It is viewed as a managerial strategy that emphasizes on joint responsibility for process quality and costs. The view that healthcare service is a *social good* implies that social responsibility is an important goal of a healthcare organization and it has a role in creating healthier communities. It is widely accepted in the field of management that progress through the application of the principles of TQM can and indeed be measured. TQM measurements vary depending on the application, and as such there exists no universally applicable set of standards. Moreover, progress through the application of TQM methods can only be measured by monitoring process improvements, and the variation of outcomes and results. It involves the review of overall organizational success. When properly implemented, it is possible to reduce waste in the processes, provide high quality services at lower costs, create a customer and employee friendly environment and provide a healthcare organization with an opportunity to compete at a higher level over a period of time.

Gaucher and Coffey (1993, p. 23) have reported about the success of the University of Michigan Medical Center's TQM process. The focus of the programme was to improve quality through meeting customer requirements and improving quality of work life. Seventeen of the 19 teams achieved significant savings through the years 1987 to 1991. Costs and benefits analysis showed that 14 of the 19 teams required negligible resources to implement their recommendations. Even with the costs of training (direct labour time, etc.), the return on investment was found to be substantial.

McLaughlin and Simpson (1999, pp. 36–37) have presented empirical evidence based on the research of Harkey and Vraciu in 1992 on the relationship between profitability and customer satisfaction in 82 Health Trust hospitals. Based on their research, the authors suggested a quality profitability model (Figure 4.4). The perception of quality by employees, patients and physicians was found to be in strong agreement and that the perception of quality, when controlled for payer mix and managed care, added to profitability. McLaughlin and Simpson (1999, pp. 36–37) concluded that it is the 'meta-relationship' that will be of great interest to the board of trustees and to the senior management, which helps in justifying CQI, based on perceived quality and profitability.

Nelson et al. (1992 cited in Kunst and Lemmink, 2000, p. 85) reported that hospital quality accounted for 17–27 per cent of the hospital earnings. Other benefits of TQM application in hospitals as per reports are: employee satisfaction, reduced costs, improved patient survival and continuity of care. McLaughlin and Simpson (1999) have further reported that the cost of poor quality can be reduced. Cost of non-conformance and waste in healthcare is estimated to be in the range of 20–40 per cent of the total cost in the American industry as reported by knowledgeable administrators.

Table 4.4 depicts the applications of TQM in healthcare and its benefits identified from the literature (excluding Indian studies).

Figure 4.4

Relationship between Costs and Quality

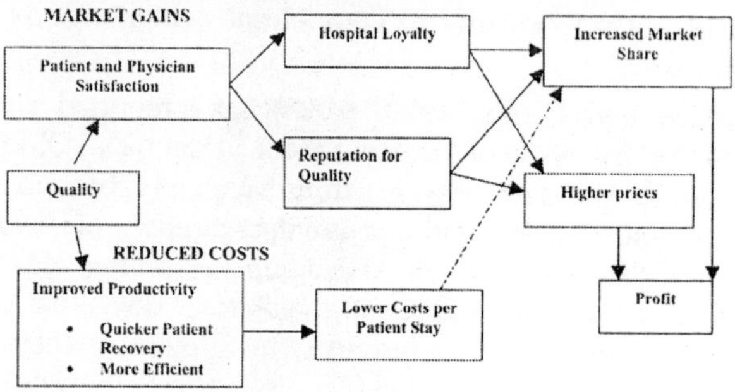

Source: McLaughlin and Simpson, 1999, p. 36.

Table 4.4

TQM Applications in Healthcare

Focus	*Application*	*Benefits*	*Reference*
Public Hospital	Hospital wide	Sustainable patient satisfaction and better interdepartmental communication.	Chow-Chua and Goh, 2002
Patient Care	Casualty and Pathology Department	Overall turnaround time (TAT) for lab tests was reduced from 45 minutes to less than 30 minutes.	Kohli et al., 1995
Patient Care	Emergency Care		
	Transportation of OB patients to OB floor	Benefits in terms of time, cost, employee morale and customer satisfaction.	Klein et al., 1998
	Availability of supplies and equipment in the emergency department		

Cont'd...

Cont'd...

	Patient admission process to hospital from Emergency Care Centre		
Patient Care	Discharge planning of chronic patients	Recommendations based on Quality Function Deployment carried out: To establish continuity of care. To strengthen the education of the patient's family. To plan further testing and referrals.	Chang and Cheng, 2003
Core Processes	Clinical Services and Business Operations	Reduction in work force planned. Established core values and behaviours. Information Systems planned and developed.	Anderson et al., 1996
Core Process Redesign	Home Health Agency	Preserve its values, reduce costs, improve service and enhance quality of customer services provided. Annual savings of $480,000	Poirier and Moran, 1998
Process Improvement	Quality of services of emergency room	Innovative use of Total Quality Management and simulation-animation technique helped determine the optimum quantity of resources necessary to successfully service a demand pattern.	Gonzalez et al., 1997
Service Delivery Improvement	Medical Photography Department-turn around time (TAT) of Fundus Fluorescein Angiograms to the Ophthalmology Department	Pilot project showed that new standards could be set for the delivery of clinical photography services focusing on the requirements of the users.	Murray, 2003

Cont'd...

Cont'd...

Admini-strative practices	Calculation and distribution of cheques	Accuracy within 3 payroll periods went up to 99.2% and finally reached 100%. HR Department saved nearly $10,000.	Moody et al., 1998
	Process of filling job vacancies by Human Resource Department	48 days eliminated from hiring cycle with an estimated profit enhancement of $ 314, 264.	
Admini-strative practices	Appointments to patients	Advancement in understanding self-organization, realization of customer-driven activity, learning that each patient needs could never be predicted and flexible methods are essential to meet each situation as it arose.	Harte and Etchart, 1997

The managerial benefits in healthcare generally come from five sources which are relevant in the context of TQM:

1. vastly increasing the capacity of the professionally dominated organization to do process analysis;
2. capturing the intellectual capital already developed by the workforce (e.g., frontline workers may know their work processes better than managers);
3. increasing the intrinsic motivation of the workforce;
4. reducing the managerial overhead necessary to induce managerial change; and
5. creating lateral linkages across highly specialized organizational units to increase effectiveness and reduce the process irresponsibility inherent in most healthcare settings. Process improvements efforts (goals, responsibilities and capacities) and quality efforts are mutually reinforcing. They lead to cost and quality improvements. Figure 4.4 shows how quality efforts and process improvement efforts are mutually reinforcing. Professionals in process improvement also contribute to the support of the quality effort and can ultimately improve both cost and quality (McLaughlin and Simpson, 1999).

In general, effectiveness of quality programmes, especially of large-scale intervention programmes is not very easy to assess and measure. Øvretveit and Gustafson (2003) have said that although some discrete quality team projects have shown to be effective, large-scale projects may not give conclusive evidence for their effectiveness. However, there is no conclusive evidence that there are no benefits and that those resources are being wasted. Measuring quality in healthcare is very complex, for instance, readmission to the hospital as a quality indicator is still debatable. Clarke (2004) has commented that whether a patient is readmitted or not is surely less important than whether he or she has a satisfactory outcome of the index of hospital stay, measured using valid and reliable indicators of health status or quality of life. In fact, owing to the nature of dynamicity of organizations and changing nature of programmes, making assessments of programmes is difficult if not impossible. For successful implementation of TQM, the critical factors have to be thoroughly understood so that managerial actions, behaviours and strategies can focus on those factors for implementation.

Summary

Managing the total quality of healthcare services is gaining ground in the hospital sector. The literature review closely examined the concepts, issues, advantages, applications and general framework of TQM in healthcare. The chapter briefly discussed the contributions of 'quality gurus' such as Deming, Juran, Feigenbaum, Crosby and Ishikawa in general. Specific contributions of healthcare quality by Donabedian, Berwick, McGlaughlin, Kaluzny and Simpson were closely examined. The discussion led to understanding the close linkages of cost, quality and process enhancements in healthcare services. The applications and advantages of implementation of TQM in healthcare services were reviewed and discussed in the chapter. Though studying of effects of TQM in dynamic and complex situations such as in hospitals is very difficult, it is not impossible. Literature shows that continuous quality improvement effects based on philosophical, structural and healthcare elements would lead to sustainable improvements in quality, processes enhancements and cost.

Research Insights

- TQM approach consists of application of selected quality management techniques throughout the organization with the aim to increase profitability through customer focus.
- TQM is known to work in healthcare settings and has shown significant advantages. Based on literature review, a number of advantages are observed: customer satisfaction, employee morale, perceptions of quality, profitability, improved outcomes, operational efficiencies and effectiveness (Gaucher and Coffey, 1993; Kohli et al., 1995; Anderson et al., 1996; Klein et al., 1998; Moody et al., 1998; Bharat et al., 1999; McLaughlin and Simpson, 1999; Singhal et al., 2000; Chow-Chua and Goh, 2002; Chang and Cheng, 2003).
- For effective implementation of TQM in an organization, it is important to identify critical quality management strategies. Such 'critical success factors or strategies' correspond to the drivers of quality performance (Kanji and Sa, 2003).
- Operational measures of quality management in terms of certain critical factors would be useful to both decision-makers and researchers. Decision-makers need to know the status and level of variables of quality management that can be effectively controlled in order to achieve high quality. The researchers can use such measures to understand quality management practices much better and build theories and models that relate to critical factors of quality management in an organization.
- It provides unique advantages over quality assurance activities by facilitating an organizational culture of quality, learning and continuous improvement.

5

Quality Management of Healthcare Services in India

Demand for healthcare services is related to population size, life expectancy and purchasing power. Potential demand for services is very promising in India based on all these factors. The health of the nation is a key issue in public policy-making and implementation through deployment of huge resources. At the national level, key issues of quality, namely, availability, accessibility, affordability, efficiency and effectiveness have been debated by policy makers, healthcare providers, healthcare managers and academia.

This chapter discusses the quality management of Indian healthcare briefly. This review includes the quality initiatives taken by both government and private-sector healthcare providers. Also, the latest trends in quality management practices in terms of NABH/ISO certification and implementation of TQM principles for achieving high quality among healthcare organizations are examined. Finally, research gaps in TQS in healthcare literature in India are identified.

Growth of Healthcare Sector in India

The Indian economy has grown at a steady level and so has the healthcare industry over the last two decades. In the last five decades, a vast healthcare infrastructure and manpower at primary, secondary and tertiary care in government, voluntary, private and corporate sector has been built up. Currently, private-sector health services range from those provided by large corporate hospitals, smaller hospitals, nursing homes and clinics run by qualified personnel. However, there is an imbalance in the distribution, with the bulk of services located in urban areas and dominated by the private sector. Figure 5.1 shows broad categories of demand and supply of healthcare services in India. There is no systematic planning and monitoring of the healthcare delivery at the state level and health services continue to be supply-pushed than demand-driven. Presently, the Indian health expenditure accounts for 5.2 per cent of its GDP; in fact, public health investment has declined from 1.3 per cent of GDP to 0.9 per cent by the year 2001. Considering the health needs of the people, our National Health Policy (2002) envisages an increase in public health spending from the present 0.9 per cent of GDP to 2 per cent by the year 2010.

Figure 5.1

Demand and Supply of Healthcare Services in India

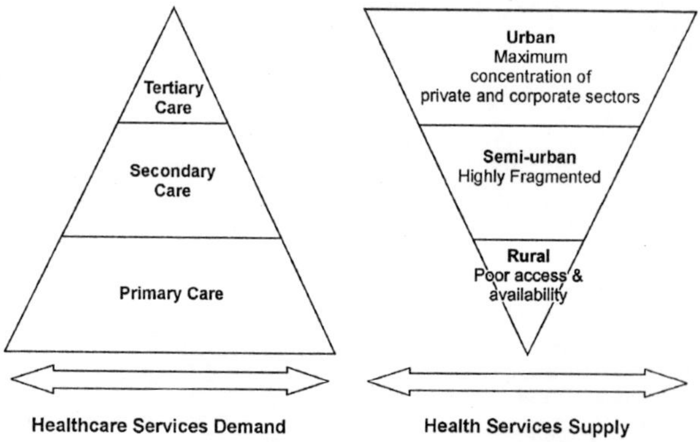

Out of the total health expenditure, 17 per cent comes from taxation, 1 per cent from Employees' State Insurance Scheme (ESIS), 14 per cent from private insurance sector and 68 per cent from out-of-pocket expenses. It is estimated that for every one rupee spent by the government only 10 per cent goes to the consumer. In general, our health services capacity is much lower than the WHO norms.

The increase in affluence among the middle class which is fast growing and estimated to be about 300 million is creating a demand for higher standards of care. In general, multi-speciality private hospitals are preferred for treatments even when the person has to bear the costs himself or herself. In the period between 1993–94 and 2001–02, the aggregate household expenditure on health services has increased at an annual compounded rate of 9.3 per cent (Ernst and Young, 2003). In addition to the demands of high quality care among those who can afford, increased information dissemination and consumerism have led to more demands. For instance, healthcare services grievances are under the purview of Consumer Protection Act; recently, the Supreme Court has held that the services rendered by the Railway Hospitals in the country would come under consumer courts to enable consumers to redress their grievances for deficiencies in services (*The Hindu,* 2005).

Nandraj et al. (2001) have reported that 60–70 per cent of outpatient cases and 40–50 per cent of hospital in-patients are managed in the private for-profit sector. The scale of operations of hospitals is not very clear in India. A total of 30,000 hospitals and 1,000,000 beds are estimated to be available (Ramani and Mavalankar, 2005). It is estimated that the private sector accounts for nearly 56 to 67 per cent of the total number of hospitals and 30 to 33 per cent of hospital beds (Phadke, 1993; Nandraj et al., 2001; Ramani and Mavalankar, 2005). Private sector also accounts for over 60 per cent of the five million doctors in the country (Ramani and Mavalankar, 2005). It is one of the highest levels of direct doctor-to-patient or hospital-to-patient transactions in Asia.

As stated earlier, private-sector health services in India range from those provided by large corporate hospitals, smaller hospitals/nursing homes and clinics/dispensaries run by qualified practitioners and services provided by unqualified persons. A majority of the private-sector hospitals are small establishments; 85 per cent of them have less than 25 beds with a average bed strength of 10 beds. Private tertiary care institutions providing speciality and super-speciality care account for only one to two per cent of the total number of institutions while corporate hospitals constitute less than one per cent.

Based on the analysis of issues and challenges of the Indian healthcare industry, the following driving factors for quality initiatives were identified:

- *A disparity between demand and supply of healthcare services* has underscored the need to address the quality issues in terms of availability, access, affordability and equity of quality in healthcare in India.
- The demands on the health system are adversely affected by *demographic factors* of growing population, large number of elderly people and poverty. *The epidemiological trends* and 'disease burden' including the HIV/AIDS, communicable and non-communicable diseases have led to renewed efforts in ensuring medical care to all. Lifestyle diseases further compound the problems of low capacity and availability of the existing healthcare delivery system.
- *Accreditation and effective quality management mechanisms in hospitals* are extremely *limited* and *emerging only recently* in India. Existing regulatory mechanisms such as licensing of medical professionals, MCI regulations for medical college hospitals and accreditation have not been effective enough for ensuring high quality of clinical care and services at the hospital level.
- Hospital administrators are interested in formalizing quality management programmes because of increasing *patient awareness, consumer group activism* and *litigation.*
- Demand for quality services is increasing among the *middle class due to awareness and affordability factors.*
- *As the private health insurance sector is growing,* the hospitals and clinics have to ensure quality of care and need more formalized reporting on quality indicators in order to streamline the claims, fees structure, etc.
- *New opportunities for growth* of private/corporate hospitals are triggered by medical tourism and the flow of revenues expected by treating foreign patients.

Hospitals are complex organizations with multiple services offered and it is important to involve everyone in managing quality. In general, the areas of productivity and efficiency are very crucial to healthcare delivery systems. Berman and Eliya (1993) have highlighted the role of government policies in influencing the development of private services in the developing countries. They have said that the quality aspects of technical care are least likely to be guaranteed through market forces. Since technical quality is least subject to evaluation by consumers, licensing and regulation are the most important mechanisms. Even when such regulations exist, enforcement has not been effective. The authors have suggested that the licensing of facilities can be made contingent up on suitable levels of quality of basic amenities, staffing and service. Quality in terms of clinical outcomes is much more difficult to assess and regulate. The lack of an effective healthcare system in India is now jarring, especially in non-urban areas, where there is a high incidence of infectious, communicable diseases and high infant mortality. Despite huge investments over many years, Indian public-sector health infrastructure is neither adequate and well managed nor sensitive. They have concluded that the role of the Government is essential to ensure a minimum baseline service of healthcare through regulation and accreditation.

Regulation and Accreditation of Healthcare Services in India

Medical training regulation, professional standards, rules for hospital waste management, clinical laboratory accreditation and consumer protection act are described here. The discussion focuses on only those regulations that are directly related to clinical care and to consumers.

- *Medical training regulation* is quite well established in India. Medical Council of India (MCI) is a statutory body, concerning the quality of medical education and for ensuring an environment conducive to learning in the teaching hospitals. In practice, it is reportedly inactive and ineffective in curbing irrational practices and malpractices (Phadke, 1993). Accreditation of hospitals by the National Board of Examinations by the Government of India (Ministry of Health and Family Welfare) for conducting post-graduate and fellowship programmes in super speciality areas is mandated.

- One way of ensuring high level of technical quality of care is through setting standards and monitoring by professional associations. Indian Medical Association (IMA) is a voluntary body for setting professional standards and for licensing and registering of medical and surgical professionals. However, IMA does not mandate renewal of registrations based on continuing medical education (CME) credits for professionals which is a standard practice in many countries. Comparing CME requirements from across the world, the USA has the most stringent requirement with their state medical boards requiring from 12 hours (state of Alabama) to 50 hours (several states) of CME per year for license re-registration. Austria has made CME certificate over a three year cycle mandatory since 2001. Netherlands has introduced re-registration with a five year interval required from 2003. Annual revalidation system of all licensed practitioners was made mandatory in December 2004, but is now under review in the UK. In India, MCI has proposed an annual continuing education (CME) but the government favours registration every five years. The doctors' opinions are divided on this and the cost of revalidation is a contentious issue (Mukherjee, 2005).
- Hospital waste management and proper disposal of biomedical waste is not only important for keeping the hospital employees, patients, patient families, etc. safe, but it is also a major environmental and community safety issue. The GoI gazette notification of Bio-Medical Waste Management and Handling Rules of 1998 established a deadline for hospitals having 500 beds and above to have waste treatment in place by 30th June 2000. Many hospitals, especially the large ones, have begun to implement the waste management programmes. The State and the Central Pollution Control Boards are a part of the regulatory authority in terms of implementation.
- Clinical Establishments Bill was passed in 2010 which mandates that all the clinical establishments such as hospitals and clinics including single-doctor establishments, with or without beds be registered. Also, all the

clinical establishments dealing with all recognized systems of medicines or treatment such as allopathy, ayurveda, unani, siddha and homoeopathy (Ayush) should be registered as per the provisions of the Bill. The Bill also proposes a multi-member National Council for Clinical Establishments to classify, determine and develop standards of clinical establishments and also to compile and publish national register of such establishments. Since the bill is passed very recently, assessing its impact on quality of hospital services will take a long time to come.

- From the consumer point of view, medical services come under the Consumer Protection Act and grievances of medical neglect by the hospitals or healthcare providers are addressed through this.
- National Accreditation Board for Laboratories (NABL, Department of Science and Technology, India) has developed ISO: 15189: 2000 standards for evaluation of quality of work and competency of medical laboratories effective from 1st June 2005. Earlier, ISO: 17025: 1999 were available for all general laboratories. The accreditation is voluntary and expensive. With an estimated one million clinical diagnostic laboratories in India, hardly 25,000 are reported to have a fair level of instrumentation and qualified staff as per the requirements.
- National Accreditation Board for Hospitals (NABH) under the Quality Council of India became operational for accrediting in 2005.

In general, the healthcare regulatory mechanisms are inadequate to ensure high quality of services in India. Even though the legislations are on their way along with accreditation, most of them are quite recent compared to the emergence of organized healthcare systems in India. The factors that contribute to the poor quality of services offered by the private sector are lack of monitoring by authorities, outdated and inadequate legislation, and the inability or failure of the government to enforce existing regulations (Nandraj, 1994; Bhat, 1996; Jesani, 1996). The studies also indicated that professional bodies, whether sanctioned by the government or voluntary medical associations, have not played a significant role in improving the private practice, especially individual practitioners and hospitals. Study by Nandraj et al. (1999) indicated that various stakeholders of hospitals in Mumbai were in favour of an accreditation system for private hospitals. With the rapid growth of private sector in India, the government has to increasingly play a complex role of being a competitor to, catalyst for and regulator of private initiatives, as it in itself cannot provide services for everybody given its limited funds. Developments in setting up of accreditation for hospitals are discussed in the next section.

Accreditation and certification for hospitals is a recent phenomenon in India. Quality has become a competitive strategy; the private sector hospitals have increasingly started looking for external certification. Hospitals have started obtaining ISO, NABH and JCI certifications in an effort to improve systems and processes for quality. Though, at this time, it can be pointed out that the hospital certification is more of a 'marketing strategy'. For instance, JCI accreditation is one of the strategies for attracting international customers/medical tourism. Nevertheless, they are very useful to establish quality levels previously not seen in India. Table 5.1 traces the trends in felt needs among the professionals for need for accreditation of hospitals in India and Table 5.2 gives the number of hospitals accredited so far.

Table 5.1

Changing Scenes of Establishment of Accreditation in India

Time Period	*Quality Management System*	*Need for Accreditation*
1980s	Doctor knows the 'best'; QMS is more of an industrial requirement and healthcare does not require	Not felt
1990s	'A New fad'; 'Let us try'; 'May be it will work, it works in other countries'	We need! But we are not sure if it can work for Indian healthcare sector
Mid 2000 onwards	Good for setting up standard systems and processes; hospitals will benefit	Works as a good marketing tool; hospitals need it urgently

NABH – The much needed Quality Standards for Healthcare in India!

National Accreditation Board for Hospitals and Healthcare Providers (NABH) was set up under Quality Council of India and became operational in 2005. The NABH standards provide a framework for quality assurance and quality improvement, while focusing on patient safety and quality of care. Specific accreditation standards are available for hospitals, small healthcare organizations, blood banks, PHCs, AYUSH Hospitals and so on. National Accreditation Board for Laboratories (NABL) standards is also available for laboratories specific to healthcare. NABH was developed using multiple information sources such as Scientific Literature and Research findings, JCI Standards, UK Healthcare Quality Standards, Thailand Standards, AHA Draft Standards, JCI Survey compliance data, ISO 9001–2000 and inputs from field experts and key stakeholders.

The main focus areas of NABH accreditation are:

- Patient and staff rights and benefits
- Patient and staff safety
- Control and prevention of infections in hospitals
- Risk management across the hospital
- Practising good patient care protocols, e.g., special care for vulnerable groups, critically ill patients
- Competencies in clinical as well as managerial practices
- Better and controlled clinical outcome and thus improving the overall functioning of the hospital

NABH standards have ten chapters incorporating 100 standards and 514 objective elements. Ten specific areas are:

1. Access, Assessment and Continuity of Care (AAC)
2. Care of Patient (COP)
3. Management of Medication (MOM)
4. Patient Right and Education (PRE)
5. Hospital Infection Control (HIC)
6. Continuous Quality Improvement (CQI)
7. Responsibility of Management (ROM)
8. Facility Management and Safety (FMS)
9. Human Resource Management (HRM)
10. Information Management System (IMS)

Table 5.2

Number of NABH Accredited Healthcare Organizations

Type of Organization	*Number of Organizations Accredited*
Hospitals	73
Applicant Hospitals	405
Blood Banks	27
AYUSH Hospitals	1
Medical Imaging Services	16 Applicants
Complied Medical Labs	116
Small Healthcare Organizations	7
Register PHCs	2
In-process	105

Source: 'Official Website of Quality Council of India' http://www.qcin.org/nabh/March 2011

Though private/corporate sector is responding to meet the demands of healthcare services, there is a need to address the issues of high quality of care at reasonable costs. Quality management practices at hospital level and improvement of the overall services are essential. Efficiency and effective management of hospitals as a healthcare provider and a business enterprise require a holistic approach. Indian public health system has so far remained mostly unaffected by the experience of many successful large-scale reform measures of different countries described in the previous chapter. Nine states in India have taken up health sector reforms and the results have been encouraging (GoI, 2004). It is to be noted that under National Rural Health Mission (2005) many quality initiatives to improve rural healthcare services have been put in place. The following section briefly discusses some significant public health initiatives taken up in five states (not directly under NRHM).

Quality Initiatives in Public Health in India

Located in South India, Andhra Pradesh is the fifth most populous state in India and the health status of the state is marginally higher than that of Indian national average. Owing to the problems of poor level of functioning and management of the public health system and limited financially resources Andhra Pradesh Vaidya Vidhana Parishad (APVVP) was set up to manage the district hospitals. The mission of each Parishad Hospital shall be to provide healthcare services with 'Care, Comfort and Courtesy'. The Parishad developed innovative ways of fund raising including charging user fees, the Anna Dana schemes, donations, lotteries and external assistance. Major areas chosen for improvements included infrastructure and utilities for the hospitals (such as buildings, equipment, water and electricity, toilet facilities, etc.). Quality of clinical care in terms of scientific evidence-based diagnostic services, hospital infection rates, drug availability, service attitudes of care and concern; referral services, patient satisfaction, etc. were focused. Subsequently, a number of reports on performance have indicated substantial improvements in quality. The Parishad constantly tries to improve its service levels not only in terms of accessibility, availability and utilization but also focuses on meeting the needs of the people with appropriate clinical care and service levels. Though the initiatives, reforms and actual implementation appear to be going well, there is a long way to go for achieving excellence in quality.

Tamil Nadu Medical Services Corporation (TNMSC) has implemented an excellent logistics management system in order to coordinate the activities of purchase, storage and distribution of drugs and medicines in Tamil Nadu (TNMSC, 2003). It is also certified by ISO (ISO 9001: 2001), and many states are planning to set up similar mechanisms to improve public-health services. The state of Maharashtra is implementing a project titled Maharashtra Health Systems Development (MHSDP) under the state public health department with an aim to provide quality services to patients. There are 136 project facility hospitals including community hospitals, sub-district hospitals and district hospitals. They are developing hospital performance analysis, patient satisfaction surveys, informatics, public-health databases, etc. in order to improve the overall service levels.

Karnataka has undertaken an initiative to accredit district and taluka hospitals in the state (Viswanathan, 2002b). Its task force on Health and Family Welfare has already achieved ISO certification for 30 health centres in Bangalore and has conducted a pilot project on 10 public hospitals.

Some states are also taking up innovative projects, for instance, the state of Madhya Pradesh has taken up a pilot project named Rogi Kalyan Samiti (RKS, 2003) in Indore with a committee formed to take full control of Maharaja Yashwantha Rao Hospital (MYH). The committee consists of people's representatives and some government office bearers. The goals of the project are to: enhance efficiency of doctors, arrest the deterioration of the hospitals, improve general condition of the facilities and increase in the number of patients at MYH. The results of such efforts have proven effective in enhancing utilization and efficiency of the system.

The above discussion highlighted the quality management initiatives taken up by selected public healthcare system of India. The following section identifies TQM trends in Indian hospitals from literature. There is an increasing interest in the use of TQM tools and techniques in various departments of hospitals across the country. In the last 10 years, global trends in quality management and implementation of TQM appear to have had an impact on the sector.

Total Quality Management of Hospitals in India

Recent trends in quality management in hospitals in India have been toward implementing TQM practices in order to make services more customer oriented. Evidence-based continuous improvement methods have been applied in various departments or units and for various hospital services. The studies highlight the importance of the concept of systems approach and system design. Rao and Agarwal (2003) have highlighted the problems of medical errors and patient safety as not just errors committed by individuals but the resultant of system failures. Using the concept of 'Vulnerable System Syndrome', they have argued that the inherent faults that lead to errors are a result of organizational pathologies. This represents the failure of system design and processes. Therefore, it is important to redesign systems geared to prevent, detect and minimize the effects of undesirable interaction effects of design, performance and circumstance.

Reddy et al. (2002) have argued that the strategic implementation of the 'Six Sigma' concept with complete involvement of the top management would make quality and measurement-oriented culture in the healthcare sector. The study reported on the reduction of waiting time in ultrasound department of a corporate hospital. It was achieved through the six sigma process of DMAIC (Define, Measure, Analyse, Improve and Control). In this study, developing QFD, identifying processes Critical to Quality (CTQ), customer expectation survey and DMAIC processes helped achieve reduced waiting time, procedure time and reporting time for ultrasound procedures.

Gupta (1998) studied the quality of services of Indraprastha Apollo Hospital, New Delhi and reported that quality management is guided by TQM. Quality is seen as everybody's responsibility and that everything the hospital does reflects quality. Quality management tools and techniques are implemented throughout the organization. The report highlighted the achievements in the area of Human Resource Management and Development of the hospital. Training of various groups of staff, exit interviews, 360 degree performance appraisal, etc. are carried out in order to achieve high quality of care. Risk management, quality management systems, good servicescapes, accreditation, etc. have made organization-wide implementation of quality management possible. The report identified weaknesses in the areas of measurement, data analysis and information integration in the hospital. Subsequently, Indraprastha Apollo has obtained JCI accreditation.

At the hospital level, the case example of Tata Main Hospital (TMH), Jamshedpur provides useful insights into the understanding of TQM implementation. TQM implementation was initiated in order to improve the perceptions of the community the hospital served (especially complaints about medical care and services), to make services cost-effective and to meet newer demands from patients (Mitra, 2001). The hospital used Tata Business Excellence Model (TBEM) based on the MBNQA model of the USA. Implementation of the TQM techniques in the hospital utilized Juran Institute's TQM approach consisting of proof of need, diagnostic journey, remedial journey and implementation and holding gains. The case study demonstrated the importance of moving beyond the ISO system in order to achieve excellence in quality. The long-term benefits included improvements in systems (various departments) and processes, streamlining human resources (reduction of workforce, training, establishing quality culture, motivation and empowerment) and fiscal discipline (and waste reduction).

Table 5.3 outlines the advantages of TQM in hospitals in India. The table indicates that majority of the studies reported are from Tata Main Hospital and therefore applicability of the MBNQA based model needs to be further researched.

Research Gaps in TQS India

Based on the literature review, the following factors of TQM implementation in hospitals in India were identified:

- Obviously, technical and medical aspects of care are important components of patient care services in terms of procedural appropriateness and risk management such as reducing hospital infection rates (Vij et al., 2001; Gupta and Kant, 2002) and improving patient care service with inputs from patients (Bharat, 1994; Bharat et al., 1998; Ray, 1999; Singhal et al., 2000; Samaddar et al., 2001). Technical competency and advanced investigation facilities were found to be important for insuring patient satisfaction (Bhardwaj et al., 2001; Verma and Sobti, 2002; Bedi et al., 2004).
- Customer focus including satisfaction, perceptions, expectations of patients (and families) as well as doctors/staff and medical officials play a crucial role in providing high quality healthcare services both in public and private healthcare organizations (Bhardwaj et al., 2001; Mahapatra et al., 2001; Verma and Sobti, 2002; Bedi et al., 2004; Rameshan and Singh, 2004). In general, majority of these studies indicated that communicating patient information, empathetic attitude and responsiveness to customer's needs was found to be important for patient satisfaction. Mahapatra et al. (2001) found corruption in public health system as the top cause of patient dissatisfaction. The study by Verma and Sobti (2002) showed that the dissatisfaction levels were higher for government hospital services than private ones. Study by Bedi et al. (2004) showed that

Table 5.3

Applications of TQM in Hospitals in India

Focus	*Application*	*Benefits*	*Reference*
Patient Care	Intensive Care Unit (two major value engineering projects comprising many small projects) on oxygen consumption and E.C.G. electrodes.	Continuous reduction in overall expenditure by eliminating waste and modified conventional practices to improve quality of care. Over a period of eight years nearly ₹ 24 lakhs were saved cumulatively.	Samaddar et al., 2001*
Patient Care	Critical Care (by defining value, finding reasons behind poor value/performance and value engineering).	Plan to identify causes for poor value, reduce costs and steps for value engineering was identified for CCU.	Ray, 1999*
Patient Care	Cardiac Care (in-hospital delays extending from arrival at hospital till thrombolytic infusion is started, i.e., door to needle time).	Streamlining hospital systems and procedures helped reduce door to needle time in thrombolytic therapy for Acute Myocardial Infarction.	Bharat et al., 1998*
Patient Care	Obstetric Unit- Perinatal Mortality Rate Reduction using root cause analysis.	Root causes were lack of on-the job training of baby's handling and resuscitation and improper protocol for high-risk pregnancy identification. 4.5 per cent cases of stillbirths were identified as preventable after an analysis over a year (Sepsis, birth asphyxia and meconium aspiration syndrome main causes of neonatal death).	Singhal et al., 2000*

Cont'd...

Cont'd...

Administrative Practices	Waiting time in outpatient services in Cardiology.	Improvement of waiting time carried out by appointment system for chronic patients, efficiency improvement of availability of doctors, introduction of practice guidelines and time management of elective procedures. After two months the average waiting time for consultation decreased from 58.6 minutes to 7.7 minutes without any additional manpower or resources.	Bharat et al., 1999*
Process Reengineering	Radiology Department	Increased efficiency of processes with overall cost reduction was possible.	Varghese, 2001
Process Improvement	Emergency Care and Patient Discharge Process	Helpful in minimizing process times.	Reddy and Acharyulu, 2003
Process Improvement	Cardiology Services	Analysis and process improvement along with patients and doctors education resulted in reduction of complications from 4.9 to 1.03 per 100 patient years, thereby improving patient safety.	Bharat et al., 1998*
Cost Minimization	Burn care (applying the concept of value engineering).	Nearly 50 per cent savings in cost of dressing materials and antibiotics were achieved.	Bharat, 1994*

Cont'd...

Cont'd...

Cost Minimization	Resource utilization in laboratory testing (Indigenous modification in the bulb holding system for two imported microscopes using low cost durable bulbs using value engineering and team effort).	Lowered cost without compromising quality.	Mishra et al., 2001*
Support Service	Hospital Kitchen	Improved patient satisfaction.	Dhanjal, 2001*
		Quality circle improved creativity of kitchen staff.	
		Improved motivation of workers.	
Support Service	Handling and Management of Hospital Waste	The implemented waste management met the statutory and legal requirement of the Government as per Bio-medical Waste Management rules 1998 and amendment of 2000.	
		A recurring income of ₹ 1.0 Lakh per annum was generated through sale of non-hazardous wastes.	Das et al., 2001*

*The studies were carried out at Tata Main Hospital, Jamshedpur, India.

patient expectations were higher for tertiary-care services than secondary-care services.

- Hospitals are incorporating process management as a very important managerial system to improve technical/medical care provided to patients (Varghese, 2001; Reddy and Acharyulu, 2003). Some studies reported the success of process management of support services (Das et al., 2001; Dhanjal, 2001).
- It is established that the servicescapes and physical infrastructure of hospitals are important criteria to ensure smooth flow and integration of various services within a hospital, which contribute to patient satisfaction and healing (Kant and Gupta, 2002). Facility tangibles such as utilities and infrastructure such as water supply, fans, lights, cleanliness were found to be important (Bhardwaj, 2001; Verma and Sobti, 2002; Bedi et al., 2004; Rameshan and Singh, 2004).
- Role of human resource management and development in quality services is often recognized as one of the most important criteria. Training, multi-skilling, service culture, performance appraisal and reward mechanisms have been identified as focus areas (Gupta, 1998; Arya et al., 2003).
- Importance of administrative practices to reduce waiting time, to integrate processes and for continuous improvement in order to achieve total quality is highlighted (Bharat et al., 1999).
- Hospital-wide implementation of TQM practices at Tata Main Hospital in Jamshedpur has been found to be successful. This strengthens the usefulness of MBNQA's seven criteria on which TBEM model is based. The criteria of Leadership, Strategic Planning, Customer and Market Focus, Measurement, Analysis and Knowledge Management, Human Resource Focus, Process Management and Business Results were found effective in organization-wide TQM implementation (Mitra, 2001; Sahni, 2001). The analysis of TQM implementation indicates that establishment of *service culture* is very important for hospitals.

Further, from the basis of websites of major hospitals, it can be said that Apollo Group of Hospitals; Manipal Hospital, Bangalore; Shankarnetralaya, Chennai; etc., use TQM-based Quality Management Systems. Though the above studies support the advantages of TQM practices, the level of implementation of various factors and their criticality is not researched and confirmed by systematic studies at multi-facility (hospitals) levels. Such research would provide specific directions to hospitals that are interested in establishing Total Quality Services (TQS).

The above discussion establishes the fact that the hospitals are initiating a number quality management practices and systems; however, research in TQS implementation is in its nascent stage in hospitals in India. Though a number of studies reported above identified the advantage of TQM in a healthcare setting in different departments or units, literature on organization-wide implementation is limited. Critical factors research for TQS was carried out by Sureshchandar et al. (2001a, b) in India on the banking services. The study indicated that servicescapes and service culture are essential to services, whereas MBNQA criteria do not include it as separate criteria. The authors have further recommended research on TQS in healthcare organizations with necessary modifications. The above literature review clearly indicates a need for identification and validation of TQS constructs for hospitals in India. Such a framework (and hence the testing instrument associated with measuring scales) of TQS constructs would give specific directions for hospital managers to operationalize the principles of TQM effectively.

Summary

This chapter examined the need for quality initiatives of Indian healthcare sector. Professional management of hospitals is becoming important in order to enhance the efficiency and effectiveness of the services. In general, regulatory mechanisms in India are quite weak and accreditation schemes for hospitals are an emerging area. Quality of many public and private healthcare services is rather questionable and some state government reforms are starting to address the issues of quality. At the same time, major high-tech hospitals, many of them private, are providing high quality of care and are well known for superior quality of medical professionals. Many of these large hospitals are setting a number of quality systems in place, obtaining ISO certification and hospital rating by commercial agencies, improving infrastructure, technological capabilities, etc. in order to improve the quality of services. Industry leaders are showing a keen interest in achieving high quality through applications of TQM principles. The literature review clearly indicated that hospitals are focusing on improving technical and medical aspects of care, customer satisfaction, process management, servicescapes and hospital infrastructure facilities, human resources management and training, and administrative practices. Measurement of results of hospital-wide TQM applications is very limited and research in the area of critical success factors for TQS is lacking in the Indian healthcare context. Development of a framework of TQS critical factors would fill the research gaps. Such a framework would be useful for decision-makers and healthcare managers for developing appropriate strategies for measurement and implementation of quality management strategies holistically. Also, such an effort would contribute to theory building in management research areas of TQS in healthcare.

6

Research on Quality Dimensions for TQS Implementation

The previous chapters examined the need for quality initiatives in healthcare, core issues in quality, assurance mechanisms and established that application of TQM in healthcare is effective. It is seen that TQM implementation in hospitals could adapt the basic philosophical and structural elements. However, the service aspects and the technical clinical/healthcare aspects have to be incorporated. This would mean that we could identify the approach as 'Total Quality Service' (TQS) and that the implementation strategy would address quality concerns of various stakeholders. Deriving from 'constructivism' approach, application of various quality dimensions or constructs would lead to total quality. This chapter examines research on quality dimensions for TQS implementation.

The hospitals are complex organizations with bureaucratic and highly departmentalized and functional-hierarchical structures. Gupta (1995) has reported that the health services sector is using quality management extensively. Service quality management basically extends the standard of quality, which people expect in clinical care into every aspect of hospital services. It involves a pervasive, across the board integration of quality care and quality of performance in everything a hospital does. This could be achieved by applying critical dimensions of quality. Critical dimensions in turn could be identified if we understood why organizations fail to implement TQM successfully.

Barriers to Implementation of Effective Quality Management

Gaucher and Coffey (1993, pp. 40–42) have identified general barriers to quality and quality improvement efforts in healthcare. They are: lack of common direction (common direction as described by statements of values, vision, mission, etc.); loss of key leaders who are committed to the philosophy of TQM in the organization; poor communication among various stakeholders of the organization; too many steps in a process; dysfunctional culture which does not encourage innovations, creativity and empowerment; and lack of integration and balance. Successful TQM requires a structure which minimizes the layers of management, empowers employees, enhances communication and fosters creativity in hospitals (Short and Rahim, 1995). The other problems identified by authors are: the unique relationship hospitals have with physicians; professional autonomy; conflict between hospital management philosophies; existing quality assurance programme and union management relationship.

Based on the literature review, Zabada et al. (1998) have identified that healthcare organizations are inward looking, they tend to focus more on the needs of care-givers and professionals than on the needs of external customers; large hospitals are organized on a hierarchical basis with bureaucratic cultures which are resistant to employee empowerment; lack of senior management commitment to TQM, etc. A vast majority of applications of TQM in many fields have been in the areas of greatest strategic priority, but in healthcare the applications have been to provide administrative support to patient care rather than addressing all areas of activities including the clinical processes which forms the core activity of hospitals. Initially, implementation of TQM in hospitals has always been met with resistance from physicians: "they feel that they have always provided the best care". A number of studies have identified obstacles for proper implementation of TQM which are summarized in Table 6.1.

However, such obstacles have been successfully overcome and a number of applications in healthcare settings and hospitals have proved that TQM can work in healthcare. In fact, Short and Rahim (1995) have stressed that the traditional focus of technical quality inherent in healthcare can be extended to include overall services to achieve excellence through adaptation of TQM principles.

Table 6.1

Barriers to TQM Implementation in Hospitals

(Gaucher and Coffey, 1993, p. 21; Short and Rahim, 1995; Aggarwal and Zairi, 1997; Nwabueze and Kanji, 1997; Zabada et al., 1998; Ennis and Harrington, 1999a, b; McLaughlin and Simpson, 1999, p. 34; Theodorakioglou and Tsiotras, 2000; Adinolfi, 2003; Kanji and SÁ, 2003)

- Lack of senior management commitment
- Fuzzy or unclear purpose or mission of organization
- Short-term orientation of administrators and managers
- Limited and poor communication of the strategies and goals
- Healthcare organizations are inward looking and focus more on care-givers and professionals
- Organizational structure highly departmentalized, hierarchical and authoritative
- Bureaucratic cultures which are resistant to employee empowerment; physician autonomy and occupational sub-cultures
- Resistance by employees including physicians, nurses and other medical staff to change
- Traditional quality approach in healthcare such as too much emphasis on technical issues
- Voice of the customer not clearly understood by providers of healthcare or down played
- Lack of appropriate resources of time, trained manpower and budget for quality activities
- Lack of consistency, alignment and integration

For successful implementation of quality management in any organization, identification of quality dimensions and determination of their criticality becomes important. In the initial phase of research, TQM critical factors are extracted from the literature review. The review is discussed under the categories of perceived service quality dimensions (by Parashuraman et al., 1985 and others), role of quality awards and research on critical factors for TQM (identification and validation) in non-healthcare and healthcare settings. The literature analysis provides insights into quality management practices and in building theories and models that relate critical factors of quality management to the organization's quality environment and quality performance. Importantly, decision-makers and managers of organizations could use these measures to bring about improvement in quality.

Research on Perceived Service Quality

Research in service quality has utilized the concept of 'perceived service quality' as identified by Parasuraman et al. (1988). It is the quality of services, as perceived by the consumers, as a result of comparison of what consumers feel service firms should offer with their evaluations/perceptions of the firm's performance. Service gap model is one of the most popular models developed by Parasuraman et al. (1985). They pointed out that while a negative discrepancy between perceptions and expectations – a 'performance gap' as it is called – causes dissatisfaction, a positive discrepancy leads to consumer delight.

Service quality dimensions

Based on the research on identifying criteria critical to service quality and scale purification, Parasuraman et al. (1988) arrived at five dimensions for service quality construct:

- *Tangibles:* physical facilities, equipment, appearance of personnel.
- *Reliability:* ability to perform the promised service dependably and accurately.
- *Responsiveness:* willingness to help consumers and provide prompt service.
- *Assurance:* knowledge and courtesy of employees and their ability to inspire trust and confidence.
- *Empathy:* caring, individual attention the firm provides to its consumers.

These dimensions are related to both the service process and its outcome, but it is not always clear how. Parasuraman et al. (1988) developed a measurement instrument to facilitate the operationalization of the gaps model of service quality known as

SERVQUAL. It requires the customers to provide, on a set of 22 items relating to the five dimensions of service quality, their expectations and perceptions of the levels of services provided by an organization. On a scale of seven points, the customers indicate agreement or disagreement with pole points of 'strongly agree' and 'strongly disagree'. The perceived service quality is computed by subtracting the expectation rating from the perceptions of services provided by an organization for 22 pairs of items. In the SERVQUAL model, the perceived service quality (or gap 5) is determined by the size and the direction of the so-called internal gaps:

1. Between customer expectations and management's perception of those expectations.
2. Between management's perceptions of customer expectations and the firm's service quality specifications.
3. Between service quality specifications and actual service delivery.
4. Between actual service delivery and external communication about the service.

The SERVQUAL instrument of Parasuraman et al. (1985) had widespread applications in a variety of organizations ranging from tyre retailing, dental service, hotels, travel and tourism, car servicing, business schools, hospitality, higher education, business-to-business partners, accounting firms, architectural services, recreational services, hospitals, airline catering, banking, apparel retailing and local government. Though the SERVQUAL instrument has been well appreciated for the evaluating service quality and its scale items are validated and supported by research, there are concerns about the statistical reliability of the measure. Despite widespread use, SERVQUAL has been the focus of considerable theoretical and empirical-based criticisms. The debate is about the stability of the five-factor solution and to the extent to which such broad categories can be hoped to reflect meaningful managerial themes. The other concerns are the validity of the five constructs given that the respondents are unable to consistently attribute scale items to the corresponding underlying dimensions (Mathews and Clark, 1997).

Analysing the works of many researchers, Cuganeshan et al. (1997) have identified the following problems with SERVQUAL:

- Use of difference score measures which often demonstrate poor reliability. A measure with low reliability may appear to possess discriminant validity simply due to its inherent unreliability and hence construct validity based on such discriminant validity is questionable.
- Variance restriction is shown to occur when different scores are used and in case of SERVQUAL, it will be so where expectations are consistently higher than perceptions.
- Concurrent measurement of expectations and perceptions are known to bring in favourable bias (move it upwards) on perceptions especially where initial expectations are high. Also, when the scenarios of expectations met and not met are tested (i.e., service experience) customers tend to overstate (and hence large perceived service quality gap) or understate their expectations (and hence smaller perceived service gap).

In addition to the above limitations of validity and reliability, Ruyter and Wetzels (1996) have emphasized that since the SERVQUAL approach is limited to existing products (because both experience and performance are taken into account), the quality of service innovations can hardly be measured. Additive relationships implied in the model may not be a realistic assumption. Therefore, Ruyter and Wetzels (1996) developed the integration of SERVQUAL instrument and conjoint analysis, called it as SERVCON and examined it in the context of service encounters in public transport in the Netherlands. The SERVQUAL approach was customized for the research setting, namely, Dutch Railways using attributes for operationalization of train guard activities. Three attribute levels were utilized to evaluate the services: 'better than expected', 'as expected as and worse than expected' with graded scale of 1 to 10. Conjoint analysis allows the attractiveness of a number of possible combinations of customer service elements (that are identified as important) and the ratings are used to estimate the part-worth of the individual levels of each service element. The study revealed a difference between employee and customer perceptions of service quality. Based on the results it was concluded that the differences between two actors in the service encounter could be confirmed. The problem with conjoint analysis methodology is that it allows measuring the main effects only with a limited number of combinations. The authors have also identified that interaction effects of a strong correlation between observed and estimated profile grades would provide a more precise picture of the evaluation of service quality during the service encounter. But, the procedure becomes very complex and difficult for incorporating a number of service quality attributes.

The above discussion on SERVQUAL indicates clearly that the reliability and validity of the dimensions are questionable. Also, when organizations implement innovative methodologies for organization-wide quality improvement, factors such as leadership and management commitment, training and development of employees, measurement of data and analysis for quality improvement, supplier quality management, etc. of the TQM framework are more useful. The following section discusses the empirical research literature on critical factors for TQM.

Research on Critical Factors for Total Quality Management

TQM can be studied from different approaches such as contributions from quality leaders, formal evaluations and empirical research. The research in general shows both strengths and weaknesses to offer solutions to all the problems encountered by firms although some common issues can be observed, such as management leadership, training, employees' participation, process management, planning and quality measures for continuous improvement. Taking the initial research as a basis, the critical factors of TQM found in the literature vary from one author to another, although there is a common core, formed by the following factors: customer focus, leadership, quality planning, management based on facts, continuous improvement, human resource management (involvement of all members, training, and work teams), learning process management, cooperation with suppliers and organizational awareness and concern for the social and environmental contexts.

Along with these factors from theoretical and empirical studies, there are a number of standardized quality-models used by firms as a guide for TQM implementation and self-evaluation of quality practices. The main models are the Malcolm Baldrige National Quality Award model in the USA, the European Foundation for Quality Management (EFQM) model in Europe and the Deming Prize model in Japan.

Role of Quality Awards in TQM Critical Factor Research

A number of countries have instituted National Quality Awards in order to promote and enhance quality products and services. In general, they are sponsored by government agencies to emphasize the economic fact that survival in global competition requires improvement to world-class status. Each award is based on a perceived model of TQM and they do not focus solely on product, service perfection or traditional quality management methods, but consider a wide range of management activities, behaviour and processes that influence the final offerings. Economic success of Japan and their product quality is now almost legendary. Embracement of total quality control (TQC) techniques propagated by Juran and Deming is one of the important factors for the transformation of Japan's industry's quality excellence. Widespread adoption of TQC was encouraged through the institution of Deming Prize, which was found very effective in Japan (Ghobadian and Woo, 1996). However, hospitals in Japan were bypassed by the quality revolution that literally transformed the other industry (Wocher, 1997).

There are a number of quality awards in different countries namely, Malcolm Baldrige National Quality Award (MBNQA), the European Quality Award (EQA), the UK Quality Award, Swedish Quality Award (SwQA), the New Zealand National Quality Award (NZQA), Rajiv Gandhi National Quality Award (RGNQA), Singapore Quality Award (SQA), the Canadian Awards for Excellence (CAE, the Quality Awards), Australian Quality Award (AQA), etc. There has been a great interest in comparing the quality awards and their criteria for their strengths and weaknesses (Ghobadian and Woo, 1996; Xie et al., 1998; Tan, 2002; Khoo and Tan, 2003). Most of the National Quality Awards except MBNQA have originated in the 1990s and they are still in the stage of accumulating learned experiences through assessing organizations for the awards. Table 6.2 lists the advantages and disadvantages of participating in quality awards for organizations. The broad aims of the quality awards are to:

- Increase awareness of 'quality' of products and services and that quality management would contribute to superior competitiveness.
- Encourage self-assessment of organizations based on the established criteria.
- Prompt sharing and cooperation among organizations on a range of issues to grow to better levels of functioning.
- Share information of quality practices and stimulate organizations to introduce 'quality management'.
- Help industry players understand the requirements of achieving 'quality excellence' and successful deployment of 'quality management' (Ghobadian and Woo, 1996).

Table 6.2

Advantages and Disadvantages of Participating in Quality Awards

Advantages	*Disadvantages*
• Winning an award is a symbol of 'quality excellence' for customers	• Award in itself does not guarantee future performance and excellence in quality
• Public recognition	• High levels of costs and time
• More companies follow example and implement TQM	• Fear of biased feedback doing more harm than good
• Provides benchmarks to other companies	• Defense mentality to external assessment rather than proactive attitude
• Feedback from experts help improve organizational processes further	

The MBNQA is the most researched model for TQM around the globe. This programme was established in 1987 through Public Law 100–107 for the purpose of providing American business with criteria for management of organizations to achieve the highest level of quality in performance. It is administered through the Department of Commerce's National Institute of Standards and Technology (NIST) with assistance from the American Society for Quality (ASQ). Healthcare version of MBNQA was developed in 1995 and in a pilot study the healthcare organizations did not score as well on the criteria as educational or industrial firms. In 1999, healthcare organizations became eligible for applying. Use of the Baldrige criteria is one method of incorporating the concepts and systems of TQM into the functioning of a healthcare services delivery organization (McLaughlin and Kaluzny, 1999). The criteria are very similar to those of private-sector manufacturing and Service Company awards with following exceptions:

Table 6.3

Criteria of Quality Awards

The Deming Prize	*European Quality Award*	*The Malcolm Baldrige National Quality Award*
Policy	Leadership	Leadership
Organization and its management	People Management	Strategic Planning
Education and dissemination	Policy and Strategy	Customer and Market Focus (Focus of and Satisfaction of Patients and other Stakeholders for Healthcare)
Collection, dissemination and use of information on quality	Resource Management	Information and Analysis
Analysis	Process Management	Human Resource Focus
Standardization	Employee Satisfaction	Process Management
Control	Customer Satisfaction	Business Results (Organizational Performance Results for Healthcare)
Quality assurance	Impact on Society	
Results	Business Results	
Planning for the future		

'Business Results' is replaced by 'Organizational Performance Results' category and 'Focus of and Satisfaction of Patients and Stakeholders' category replace the 'Customer and Market Focus'. Deming Prize (Japan), the European Quality Award (EQA) of Western Europe (based on European Foundation of Quality Management, EFQM) and the MBNQA of the USA have played a key role in the quality revolution. Table 6.3 gives the criteria of three important quality awards. The award criteria evolved over a period of time, e.g., MBNQA criteria and sub-criteria since established in 1987 has shifted emphasis from quality assurance to process management to quality management and now to the overall performance management in the USA.

Analysis of Literature on Critical Success Factors for TQS

The subject matter of quality management in manufacturing industry has been a matter of great interest and concern for business and academia alike. Several works have thoroughly investigated the various dimensions, techniques and organizational requirements for effective implementation of TQM. Saraph et al. (1989) conducted one of the first empirical studies to validate an instrument for integrated quality management. Total Quality Management as we have noted earlier, encompasses all systems and processes, clinical and non-clinical, with actions directed toward processes to improve the quality of all services and products for patients and all customers (Gaucher and Coffey, 1993, p. 20). This research work is an attempt to develop a measuring model for TQS hospital services based on extensive literature review, analysis and synthesis of critical factor research from TQM research in non-healthcare and healthcare environment. Such an approach would extract factors common to all organizations as systems, take into consideration the special needs of services (namely, features of service intangibility, simultaneity of production, delivery and consumption, perishability and variability) and healthcare-specific elements (for, e.g., medical records data, involvement of the medical staff governance process such as quality assurance, ethical committees, pharmacy and therapeutic committees, peer review, use of risk-adjusted outcome measures and risk management (McLaughlin and Kaluzny, 1999, pp. 8–10).

Many researchers have identified the need for investigations of measurable variables associated with each of the TQM critical factors using data inputs from large number of healthcare organizations to allow for generalizations (Adinolfi, 2003). An exploratory survey of quality practices of 31 hospitals by Lin and Clousing (1995) indicated that TQM in healthcare services is a fruitful research area. A better understanding of mechanisms and gathering of information about effects of executive participation and involvement in TQM programmes is needed. Examining the current research status of TQM in healthcare, Øvretveit and Gustafson (2003) highlighted that research in quality management programmes are difficult as healthcare organizations are very dynamic in nature and also, large-scale projects are difficult to provide conclusive evidence for TQM's effectiveness. Therefore, they have suggested that research to identify factors for successful implementation of TQM would be very useful.

The majority of factors extracted in the research studies correspond to quality award criteria, especially MBNQA. Researchers on TQM critical factors have often used Baldrige framework, as it has one of the well-accepted criteria and tested over time (Black and Porter, 1996; Flynn and Saladin, 2001). In fact, owing to specific nature of needs of healthcare services, MBNQA has come up with healthcare quality criteria with suitable modifications discussed earlier. However, measurement of organizational performance and results construct of MBNQA is not resolved (Flynn and Saladin, 2001; Meyer and Collier, 2001). Sureshchandar et al. (2001a, b) identified Servicescapes and Service Culture as critical to services quality in their TQS model but these two factors are not exclusively dealt with in MBNQA. Also, Counte and Meurer (2001) highlighted a need for more research on the increased use of criteria other than the Baldrige categories, improved measures for implementation and the use of different types of respondents from multiple organization levels. Further, general application of EQA as an evaluation instrument is debatable based on empirical research by Kunst and Lemmink (2000). Though the researchers can use the quality award criteria as a base for constructing TQM frameworks, conceptual theory building from extensive literature and expert inputs is essential in the healthcare sector.

Research Insights: Quality Awards

- All the three award criteria are prescriptive in nature but only Deming Prize clearly indicates the tools, techniques and practices, and every factor is weighted equally for contributing to organizational overall progress.
- The Deming Prize is not based on an underlying framework linking concepts, activities, processes and results together with a causality relationship but provides a list of good quality-oriented management practices. On the other hand, MBNQA and EQA attempt to model a causal relationship among different constituents of TQM.
- Counte and Mourer (2001) examined the Baldrige, King's Fund and EFQM award categories, and identified seven categories which can be considered as additional, namely, innovation, product control, contract requirements, inspection/audit and servicing.
- Many national quality awards are directly based on MBNQA and there is lack of rigorous empirical testing on the causal relationships among criteria in healthcare in different countries.
- Tan (2002) has highlighted that the *economic and social development of a country* influence the emphasis/weights given to various criteria in assessing their importance. In less developed countries, senior management commitment and leadership is emphasized but not impact on society as organizations may not be competitive.
- Quality maturity level is tied closely to its economic development and weights have to be adjusted.
- *Culture* is another factor which plays a role on the criteria selection and weights given to a particular criterion, e.g., EQA gives a higher weight to both impact on society and people management. European directors recognize the need for their companies to act within a social as well as economic context. However, in Singapore, initiatives were developed to ensure that quality systems were in line with the international standards and secured overseas recognition.
- The applicability of specific TQM methods in any enterprise is dependent on the business context and the organizational culture.

Identification of Quality Constructs of TQS in Healthcare

The literature of quality management implies that as decision-makers of an organization focus on better management of the critical factors, improvements in quality of products or services will occur and ultimately result in improved organizational performance financially as well as in customer loyalty and satisfaction. Though hospitals keep data on medical errors, mortality, morbidity rates and costs, these are not measures of organization-wide quality management. A plethora of healthcare quality literature indicates that TQM in healthcare would work and result in enhancing the organization's overall performance as a healthcare provider as well as a business enterprise.

The identification and selection of the constructs in this chapter are based on the analysis of the empirical research by Saraph et al. (1989), Ahire et al. (1996), Black and Porter (1996), Ang et al. (2000), Zhang et al. (2000) and Flynn and Saladin (2001). Sureshchandar et al. (2001b) empirically validated their TQS framework on banking services in India and constructs, service culture and servicescapes are of special interest to healthcare services also. Criticality of constructs to healthcare was further based on the empirical research by Huq (1996), Kunst and Lemmink (2000), Meyer and Collier (2001) and Chow-Chua and Goh (2002). These constructs span the entire range of activities deemed critical by the Baldrige Health Care Criteria Award (2003) along with service quality criteria of Servicescapes and Service Culture as critical to hospital services. Studies indicate that the construct 'Supplier Quality Management' is crucial to healthcare service quality, though Sureshchandar et al. (2001a, b) did not consider it in their TQS model. But, the construct is deemed critical to healthcare. The comparative analysis of all the works is given in Tables 6.4 and 6.5. The comparison is based on the scale items corresponding to the critical factor using judgemental process. The 28 dimensions of MBNQA Health Care Criteria based on Meyer and Collier's (2001) research are shown in Table 6.6.

Raja et al. (2007) arrived at a service quality model for healthcare from MBNQA, EFQM and KBEM criteria with Leadership, Process and People Management, Measurement of

Resources and Customer Satisfaction as important constructs. Naidu (2009) systematically reviewed 24 articles published internationally for factors that determine patient satisfaction and healthcare quality. She arrived at a comprehensive model with value chain actors and linkages (patient, provider and healthcare system), moderating factors (socio-demographic and contextual factors) and patient satisfaction (mostly based on SERVQUAL) which would lead to patient loyalty. Even though the model provides useful insights about interlinkages of micro-and macro-level factors, the model does not directly provide specific guidelines to management practices at the organizational level for

Quality Constructs Identified in the Present Research

The constructs can be broadly classified under three categories:

1. The dimensions that are generic to quality management of organizations belonging to different sectors but which are initially extensively practiced in the manufacturing set-up and later found valid to services including healthcare. These factors are Leadership and Management Commitment, Strategic Planning, Human Resource Management and Development, Process Management, Management of Information and Analysis, Supplier Quality Management, Customer Focus and Satisfaction and Key Results.
2. The factors that need to be specially addressed in service organizations namely Servicescapes and Service Culture.
3. The factors which are critical to healthcare organizations, namely, Healthcare Service Design, Administrative System and Social Responsibility, are included as separate factors. The Patient Care Service Design (labelled as Healthcare Service Design is this research) is recognized specifically by MBNQA healthcare criteria. Administrative System is an important part of hospitals in terms of integrating various functions of a hospital and providing basic support to all operations. Social Responsibility is addressed in some models (e.g., EQA identifies it as a separate factor). But healthcare being a social good and a basic right of individuals, Social Responsibility warrants its inclusion as a separate factor.

achieving high quality services. Further, in the Indian sub-continent context, Andaleeb et al. (2007) found that service orientation of doctors is an important factor and that foreign doctors were rated higher than the local doctors by patients in Bangladesh. A study on culture and quality care perception carried out by Rabbani et al. (2009) in Pakistan highlighted the importance of people management aspects in achieving high quality care. The study implied the role of participatory and open culture for achieving quality and the need for leadership to better utilize suggestions for improving quality care, strengthening the process of information and analysis, and encouraging rewards and recognition for employees.

After analysis and synthesis of quality management literature, it is found that 13 construct structures for TQS in healthcare organizations would adequately address all the areas of quality performance and strategies (Manjunath et al., 2007). They are:

1. Leadership and Management Commitment,
2. Strategic Planning,
3. Human Resource Management and Development,
4. Healthcare Service Design and Improvement,
5. Process Management,
6. Service Culture,
7. Servicescapes,
8. Administrative System,
9. Measurement, Information and Analysis,
10. Supplier Quality Management,
11. Customer Focus and Satisfaction,
12. Key Results, and
13. Social Responsibility.

Table 6.4
Critical Factors of TQM

Author(s)	*Location*	*Industry*[1]	*Method*[2]	*Respondents*	*Reliability*	*Validity*	*No. of Factors*	*Questions/ Items*
Saraph, Benson and Schroeder (1989)	US	M	S	162 general managers and quality managers of 89 divisions	Y	Y	8	78
Ahire, Golhar, and Waller (1996)	US	M	S	371 plant managers	Y	Y	12	60
Black and Porter (1996)	Europe	M	S	204 quality/senior managers from member organizations of EFQM	Y	Y	10 (based on Baldrige non-result criteria)	32 (items based on Baldrige Model)
Huq (1996)	US	S-H	I	About 24 TQM personnel	N.A.	N.A.	10 quality dimensions involving management issues; 8 control and implementation. (Causal relationships-empirical evidence)	N.A.
Flynn and Saladin (2001)	US, Germany, Japan, England and Italy	M	S	4264 respondents (most qualified) in 164 plants from a list of World Class Manufacturing Database, Round II	Y	Y	7 MBNQA Criteria (Validating theoretical model)	67

Cont'd...

Cont'd...

Zhang et al. (2000)	China	M	S	Senior (or quality) managers from 212 companies	Y	Y	11	78
Kunst and Lemmink (2000)	Spain, German and Netherlands	S-H	S	General managers or quality managers of 227 hospitals	Y	Y	8 EQA Criteria	36
Meyer and Collier (2001)	US	S-H	S	Senior quality managers of 228 hospitals	Y	Y	7 MBNQA Healthcare Criteria with 28 dimensions	115
Sureshchandar, Rajendran and Anantharaman (2001)	India	S-G	S	248 executives from 43 banks	Y	Y	12	126
Chow-Chua and Goh (2002)	Singapore	S-H	CS	Reporting; mainly of quality steering committee	N.A.	N.A.	7 Singapore Quality Award Criteria	N.A.

1 = M – Manufacturing, S-H – Service Healthcare, S-G – Service General

2 = S – Survey; I – Interview; CS – Case Study

Table 6.5

Comparison of 13 Constructs from the Present Research to Critical Factors of TQM by Various Authors

Critical Factors	*Saraph, Benson and Schroeder (1989)[M]*	*Ahire, Golhar, and Waller (1996)[M]*	*Black and Porter (1996)[M]*	*Huq (1996)[1]*	*Flynn and Saladin (2001)*	*Zhang et al. (2000)[M]*	*Kunst and Lemmink (2000)*	*Meyer and Collier (2001)[2]*	*Sureshchandar, Rajendran and Anantharaman (2001)[S]*	*Chow-Chua and Goh (2002)[3]*
Leadership and Management Commitment	Top Manage-ment Leadership	Top Management Commitment	Strategic Quality Management	Management Commitment Commitment to Continuous Improvement	Leader-ship	Leadership	Leadership	Leadership	Top Management Commitment and Visionary Leadership	Leadership and Quality Culture
Strategic Management		Benchmark-ing		Quality Mission Statement	Strategic Planning	Vision and Plan Statement	Policy and Strategy	Strategic Planning	Benchmarking Continuous Improvement	Strategic Planning
Human Resource Planning, Training and Development	Employee Relations Training	Employee Training Employee Empower-ment Employee Involvement	People and Customer Management	Familiarity with TQM Education and Training Performance Appraisal System Worker Empowerment	Human Resource Focus	Education and Training Employee Participation Recognition and Reward	Personnel Manage-ment	Human Resource Develop-ment and Manage-ment	Human Resource Management Union Intervention	Human Resource Develop-ment and Manage-ment

Cont'd...

Cont'd...

Service (or Product) Design (Patient Care Services in Healthcare)	Product Design	Design Quality Management	External Interface Management		Product Design		Patient Healthcare Design and Services	Technical System		
Process Management	Process Management		Operational Quality Planning	Causes of quality variation Problem-solving approach	Process Management	Process Control and Improvement	Process Management	Part of HRM	(Part of Technical System)	Management of Process Quality
Service Culture (or Quality Culture for Manufacturing Industry)		Corporate Quality Culture	Remove barriers for consensus Communications in Company Service Culture							
Servicescapes (Physical infrastructure)	Servicescapes									
Administrative System			Comparison of planned with actual performance	(Part included in Process Management)		(Part included in Process Management)				

Cont'd...

Cont'd...

Measurement, Information and Analysis	Quality Data Reporting Role of Quality Depart-ment	Internal Quality Information Usage SPC Usage	Quality Improvement Measurement Systems Team Work Structures Communicat-ion Improvement Information	Measures of costs of quality Statistical Evidence of Quality Quality Circles/Teams	Informa-tion and Analysis	Evaluation Quality System Improvement	Resource Manage-ment	Information and Analysis	Information and Analysis System	Use of Information and Analysis
Supplier Quality Management	Supplier Quality Manage-ment	Supplier Quality Management Supplier Performance	Supplier Partnerships	Supplier Development		Supplier Quality Manage-ment		(Part of patient care design and services)		
Customer Focus and Satisfaction		Customer Focus	Customer Satisfaction Orientation	Customer Focus Customer Feedback-Vehicles used	Customer and Market Focus	Customer Focus	Customer Satisfaction Employee Satisfa-ction	Focus on and satisfaction of patients and other stakeholders	Customer Focus	Customer Focus and Satisfaction
Key Results		Product Quality		Business Results		Organi-zational Performance Results	Employee Satisfaction	Quality Operational Results		

Cont'd...

Cont'd...

Social Responsibility		(Part of Leadership)	Effect on Society	(Part of Leader-ship)	Social Respon-sibility

[1]=the study arrived at two sets of dimensions: The first 10 include dimensions of Quality Management and the next eight include dimensions of Quality Control and Implementation.

[2]=the factor analysis of Baldrige Criteria based on empirical research yielded a total of 28 dimensions (the details of the 28 dimensions are given in Table).

[3]=the researchers used Singapore Quality Award Criteria and arrived at an integrated model using Kaplan's Business Score Card for performance evaluation.

[M]=Manufacturing.

[S]=Service.

Table 6.6

Baldrige Health Care Pilot Criteria: 28 Dimensions (Meyer and Collier, 2001)

Leadership	• Senior executive and healthcare staff leadership • Leadership system and organization • Public responsibility and citizenship
Measurement Analysis and Knowledge Management	• Management of information and data • Performance comparisons and benchmarking • Analysis and use of organization-level data
Strategic Planning	• Strategic development • Strategy deployment
Human Resources	• Human resource planning and evaluation • Employee/healthcare staff work systems • Employee/healthcare staff education, training and development • Employee/healthcare staff well-being and satisfaction
Patient Healthcare Design and Services	• Design and introduction of patient healthcare services • Delivery of patient healthcare • Patient care support services design and delivery • Community health services design and delivery • Administrative and business operations management • Supplier performance management
Organization Performance Results	• Patient care results • Patient care support services results • Community health services results • Administrative, business and supplier results • Accreditation and assessment results
Customer Focus	• Patient and healthcare market knowledge • Patient/stakeholder relationship management • Patient/stakeholder satisfaction determination • Patient/stakeholder satisfaction results • Patient/stakeholder satisfaction comparison

Research Gaps in Critical Factor Research in Healthcare

Based on the above literature review, the following research gaps are identified in the area of critical factors for TQM in healthcare:

- Identification and validation of TQM critical factors in the manufacturing sector is quite well established (Saraph et al., 1989; Ahire et al., 1996; Black and Porter, 1996; Ang et al., 2000; Zhang et al., 2000). In general, top management commitment and leadership, customer focus, information and analysis, training, supplier management, process management, teamwork, product and service design, process control, benchmarking, continuous improvement, employee empowerment, quality assurance, social responsibility and employee satisfaction are the most commonly extracted factors (Sila and Ebrahimpour, 2003). However, the applicability and transferability of a generic model to different countries is debatable. Critical success factors of TQM are affected by internal and external business contexts. They are: type of sector (manufacturing or service), country's economic and social development culture, information technology, government regulations, the extent of industrialization and TQM maturity levels (Lakhe and Mohanty, 1994; Kunst and Lemmink, 2000; Tan, 2002; Tari, 2002; Sila and Ebrahimpour, 2003). Based on empirical observations, Mandal et al. (2000) stressed that the organizational culture, technology use, and training and development factors are important in the Indian context. Therefore, there is a need for further research on critical factors for a developing country such as India.
- The TQM framework has to consider the service intangibility, inseparability, perishability, variability of expectations of the customers and the participatory role of customers in the service delivery. Sureshchandar et al. (2001a, b) included servicescapes and service culture in their TQS model to address the special needs of the service sector. Further, healthcare-specific elements such as epidemiological studies with insurance payments and medical records data, involvement of the medical staff governance process (quality assurance methods such as peer review, hospital acquired infection committee, audit committee), risk-adjusted outcome measures (based on severity of illness, age, etc.), cost-effective analysis, use of quality

assurance data and risk-management data have to be incorporated in the TQS for hospitals (McLaughlin and Kaluzny, 1999, pp. 8–10).

- The majority of factors extracted in the research studies correspond to quality award criteria, especially MBNQA. Researchers on TQM critical factors have often used Baldrige framework as it is well-accepted and tested over time (Black and Porter, 1996; Flynn and Saladin, 2001; Sila and Ebrahimpour, 2003). In fact, owing to the specific nature of needs of healthcare services, MBNQA has come up with healthcare quality criteria with suitable modifications. However, measurement of Organizational Performance and Results construct of MBNQA is not resolved (Flynn and Saladin, 2001; Meyer and Collier, 2001). In addition, for the Indian context, servicescapes and service culture found relevant by Sureshchandar et al. (2001a, b) are not exclusively dealt with in MBNQA. Also, Counte and Meurer (2001) identified a need for more research on criteria other than the Baldrige categories, improved measures for implementation and the use of inputs from respondents in multiple organization levels.
- General application of EQA as an evaluation instrument is debatable based on the empirical research by Kunst and Lemmink (2000). Also, Counte and Meurer (2001) stressed the need to develop conceptual TQS criteria so that organizations can better evaluate their quality management efforts in the healthcare sector.
- Huq (1996) arrived at a framework of TQM dimensions based on the works of the quality guru, which includes the management, control and implementation issues in TQM for hospitals. Rigorous statistical methodology for theory building was lacking in the study and a measurement instrument was not fully developed. Kanji and SÁ (2003) presented an implementation plan and measurement of quality performance to help sustain healthcare excellence; however, they did not empirically validate the model.

The above research gaps clearly indicate a need for the development of the TQS framework with associated constructs and scales that accurately capture the TQS criteria for hospitals. The quality issues, challenges and TQM applications in Indian healthcare sector is analysed in depth in the next chapter in order to facilitate the development of the TQS framework in the Indian context.

Summary

Often, healthcare organizations are seen to move from inspection-oriented quality improvement system to one that orients itself to a systematic transformation of organizational culture through a comprehensive plan involving customer focus, key-process monitoring, data-driven tools, and techniques and team empowerment. Therefore, managing the total quality of healthcare services is gaining ground. The literature review closely examined the concepts, issues, advantages, applications and general framework of TQM in healthcare. For successful implementation of TQM, the critical factors have to be thoroughly understood so that managerial actions, behaviours and strategies can focus on those factors for implementation. Several quality management models and frameworks from literature were closely examined to identify the research gaps. Barriers to TQM implementation in hospitals, research on perceived service quality, quality award criteria, TQM critical factors research from manufacturing, services and healthcare research were reviewed. A 13-construct TQS framework with associated scales that accurately captures the TQS criteria specifically for hospitals has been identified.

7

Validating Quality Constructs

Observations from Studies in Indian Hospitals

The previous chapter presented the selection and identification of 13 TQS constructs for healthcare organizations through the analysis and synthesis of literature. Two studies were undertaken to verify the appropriateness of these constructs in the Indian context. First is a case study of a hospital in which quality performance was measured using Balridge Healthcare Criteria. The second study explored the quality management practices in major hospitals in India through checklist-based surveys and interviews of hospital managers. The content validity of the constructs was verified using qualitative analysis of the results of these two studies. This chapter describes the details of the two studies, their rationale, objectives, results and inferences.

Study One

Quality Performance Measurement of a Hospital Using Baldrige Healthcare Criteria: A Case Study

The literature search and construct identification indicated that the TQS model with 13 constructs is suitable for healthcare organizations. Critical factors of quality are as much a base for implementation of TQS as measuring quality performance levels of an organization. Before going for a multi-facility survey and validation of the framework so developed, there is a need to make the TQS measuring instrument suitable for the Indian context. Exploratory qualitative research and content analysis is very useful in the area of quality management of hospitals (Øvretveit and Gustafson, 2003). This can be done through direct observation, interviews and case study research methods. A case study research using in-depth interviews of Senior Managers of a well-established major hospital was conducted. In this research work, the starting point for the researcher was to understand quality management practices and evaluate implementation levels of the case hospital. For this purpose, a well-researched Quality Award Criteria was applied to assess the quality performance levels of the case hospital.

Rationale for using MBNQA Healthcare Criteria and for Choosing the Hospital

As already discussed in the earlier chapters, many research studies on critical factors have used the Baldrige criteria (Black and Porter, 1996; Counte and Meurer, 2001; Flynn and Saladin, 2001; Meyer and Collier, 2001). The constructs selected in the present research also span the entire range of Baldrige criteria in addition to other criteria (such as servicescapes, service culture, etc.). In the Indian context, Tata Main Hospital, Jamshedpur has implemented TQM using the TBEM model on the lines of MBNQA and found it useful. Further, during the initial interviews conducted with a Senior Manager (Strategic Management) at Apollo Gleneagles Hospital, Kolkota, it was gathered that the experience with the use of MBNQA criteria and Balanced Score Card for quality management was quite useful. Therefore, Baldrige healthcare criteria were used in this exploratory case study for measuring the quality performance.

The rationale for choosing the case hospital to study quality management is owing to its superior medical facilities, high quality of care and more importantly, the willingness of the top management to participate in the study. It is the fourth hospital in the country to have obtained ISO 9002 certification. The hospital has established formal quality management programme based on the principles of TQM and strives to continuously improve the quality of services. The Chairman of the hospital has received a number of prestigious awards (including Padma Sri, a civilian award of very high order awarded by the Government of India) in recognition of his contributions in providing healthcare services to the community. Further, the hospital permitted the researcher to interview several managers including the Chairman as well as make observations in the hospital.

This 350-bed multi/super-speciality private hospital is located in a non-metro city of South India and is run by a charitable trust. The hospital was established in 1975 as a modest 40-bed hospital with a staff of three doctors and 12 nurses, now it can boast of over 20 speciality departments and a total staff of about 1,200 including 150 doctors specialized in various fields and 600 nursing staff. The hospital offers a wide range of medical and surgical speciality areas including cadaver kidney transplantation, neurosurgery, cardiac and cancer treatment facilities. All the support services of a modern super-speciality hospital including blood bank and state-of-the-art diagnostic facilities are available. The hospital is recognized by the National Board of Examinations by the Government of India (Ministry of Health and Family Welfare) for conducting post-graduate and fellowship programmes in super-speciality areas. The main challenges for the hospital are the competition from local hospitals, designing new healthcare services, offering services at affordable prices, meeting ever-growing customer demands and initiating health insurance schemes.

Method and Data Analysis

Question items corresponding to the healthcare criteria of MBNQA (2003) were used as a tool to evaluate quality at the Hospital. Eight managers were interviewed using both structured and unstructured in-depth interviews. The managerial representation included top-level management, senior consultants, clinical and non-clinical heads of departments. In general, the Senior Managers are responsible for guidance, implementation of quality initiatives and achievement of results. The Chairman, Human Resource Manager, Senior Medical Consultants, Head-House Keeping and Head-Legal participated in the study. The interview time ranged from one to one-and-half hour per person. After describing the purpose of the study, each respondent was asked the questions and answers were noted down during the interview. The respondents were asked to rate each question based on their perceptions of the hospital's quality programmes. A Likert Scale of ratings from 1 to 10 was used; with 1 being 'no quality programme in place' to 10 being 'completion of the project'. The respondents substantiated their ratings based on the current quality practices including structures, processes, outcomes and/or implementation levels. Approximately, another 8–10 hours of time was spent in the hospital visiting various departments and areas of the hospital to make observations and to gather further evidence. Relevant documents (such as brochures, hospital magazines, policy statements, etc.) were examined with the permission of the managers. During the analysis of the data, some additional inputs were sought through telephonic interviews and e-mails with the Senior Consultants.

The data analysis was carried out as indicated below:

- Respondents' ratings were averaged for each sub criteria (*R*) of MBNQA (refer to Table 7.1).
- The average rating was converted to MBNQA points with reference to its maximum points.
- MBNQA points for each sub criteria is calculated as given below:
  MBNQA points for each sub-criteria = [(*R*/10)* (Max MBNQA point)]
  where R = Average rating for each sub criteria.
  The ratings from all respondents were considered.
- Finally, MBNQA points for each sub criteria were added to give the total MBNQA points for the case hospital.

Analysis of Quality Performance Based on Baldrige Criteria

The results of averaged ratings (*R*) for each sub criteria and the MBNQA points are given in Table 7.1. This case hospital with more than 750 MBNQA points (out of 1000) is judged to be performing at golden level. The hospital has been quite successful in moving forward from ISO certification and in integrating continuous quality improvement in many areas of management.

The analysis of quality management using MBNQA criteria of the case hospital supports that committed leadership is a driver for management accountability and creation of environment for empowerment and organizational agility. The hospital has effectively implemented the leadership's vision even though it has a top-down structure at the outset. Leadership vision is 'to make the hospital a Mayo Clinic of India' and one Senior Consultant noted, "... the Chairman is a man with great foresight and intellect". Allocation of resources, setting up of systems, formal daily meetings with various level managers and proper communication indicate management commitment for continuous improvement.

Social responsibility issues are addressed through free medical camps, cataract eradication programmes and treatment at concession rates for those who cannot pay full charges. According to the Human Resource Manager, the hospital is run on the basis of 'highly reasonable ethical practice'. However, as noted by one of the Senior Consultants, high costs of medical care with advanced technology and medicines has made it difficult to balance the social equity issues and profits for a private hospital.

Strategic planning areas include setting up of high quality standards, improving organ transplant/donor availability, educating insurance companies about customizing medical insurance schemes and tapping the international market (also referred to as medical tourism), and expanding to Dubai. Strategic development process and implementation is obviously a great plus for the hospital considering its growth, positioning in the region and the range of services such as new the Cancer Centre and the success of the Cardiac Centre.

Focus on patients, other customers and markets is highlighted in the use of patient satisfaction survey and feedback forms effectively. A number of open communication channels interfacing patients/families, suppliers, community and staff are used to ensure patient satisfaction. Well-planned physical infrastructure and artefacts (brochures, website, grievance and complaint boxes on all floors) and a clean/hygienic ambience support the services. A general customer friendly environment and helpful front-desk staff further add value to the service aspects of care.

Measurement, analysis and knowledge management of medical care procedures and outcomes are given primary importance. Mortality and morbidity data analysis along with medical records, department records and summary of results are maintained. Accessibility, security and confidentiality issues of information are strictly adhered to. The data were insufficient for the interviewer to make conclusive judgements about the hospital data analysis used for performance review by senior leaders. The data analysis for various processes and a number of performance measures is rather limited due to a heavy patient load and excess work demands on the hospital staff. At this point, this is an area of weakness for the hospital; however, information technology-based Hospital Information System is being developed and necessary investments are being made toward this.

Table 7.1

MBNQA Points for the Case Hospital based on Self-Reporting by Senior Managers

Baldrige Criteria Category	*Average Score 'R' for MBNQA Sub-criteria on a Scale of 1–10*	*MBNQA Points for Case Hospital*	*Maximum MBNQA Points*
Organizational Profile	**Descriptive**	NA*	NA*
(a) Organizational Environment			
(b) Organizational Relationships			
1. Leadership		**103**	**120**
(a) Senior Leadership	9	63	70
(b) Governance and Social Responsibilities	8	40	50
2. Strategic Planning		**68**	**85**
(a) Strategy Development Process	8	32	40
(b) Strategic Objective	8	36	45

Cont'd...

Cont'd...

3. Patients/Market Focus		**68**	**85**
(a) Patient, Other Customer and Healthcare Market Knowledge	8	32	40
(b) Patient and Other Customer Relationships and Satisfaction	8	36	45
4. Measure, Analysis and Knowledge Management		**54**	**90**
(a) Performance Measurement	6	27	45
(b) Performance Analysis	6	27	45
5. Staff Focus		**78**	**85**
(a) Work Systems	9	32	35
(b) Staff Learning and Motivation	9	23	25
(c) Staff Well-Being and Satisfaction	9	23	25
6. Process Management		**68**	**85**
(a) Healthcare Processes	8	36	45
(b) Support Processes	8	32	40
7. Organizational Performance Results		**314**	**450**
(a) Healthcare Results	9	90	100
(b) Patient- and Other Customer-Focused Results	8	56	70
(c) Financial Market Results	9	63	70
(d) Staff and Work Systems	9	63	70
(e) Organizational Effectiveness Results	8	56	70
(f) Governance and Social Responsibility Results	7	49	70
	Total Points	**753**	**1000**

*Not applicable

Human resource development is judged to be highly effective based on training, continuous learning and professional development activities carried out in this hospital. Systems and procedures for recruitment (both internal and external sources) and career progression are done in letter and spirit. Customers', co-workers, and senior colleagues' feedback constitute an important component of performance appraisal, done every six months. Staff orientation, training – general skills and special skills (e.g., interpersonal skills, cardiac surgery team related), continuous medical education and continuous professional development programmes are the major efforts in training and skill development. Rewards, monetary and others (e.g., best employee of the month) are used for motivating the staff. Nursing staff attrition is reportedly more than that of doctors and the HR department tries to analyse and understand reasons, and minimize attrition through a number of benefits, such as children's educational support, training for professional development, etc. This is a major strength area for the hospital though challenges such as staff retention, motivation, transparency and procedures continue to exist. Staff counselling and support programmes are a part of staff development in addition to training and career progression.

Healthcare process management involves departmental procedures/protocols written (and documented) and key-processes monitoring. Standard operating procedures (SOPs) for emergency, laboratory, routine admissions, registrations, etc. are in place. Feedback to improve healthcare processes is an important feature. Feedback is obtained on service, technology/equipment used and treatment aspects of care. Doctors' inputs, latest information from medical journals and management inputs are used for improving the care processes. Measurement and data analysis for healthcare processes and outcomes is rather basic and needs improvement. Support processes such as pharmacy, central sterilization, diet, nutrition, etc. are very well streamlined with other processes. Safety and security processes (e.g., fire drills, security logs, disaster management team, etc.) are standardized.

Organizational performance results as per the reporting of the managers is comparable to any multi-speciality hospital in India. The hospital is reported to be a profit-making venture, however, no specific financial data were revealed. The hospital's cardio thoracic surgery centre was started three years back and achieved break-even at the end of two years. The hospital obtained 314 out of 450 MBNQA points, which reflects good performance. The customers including patients, employees and others like suppliers are highly satisfied as understood from the loyalty and work performance results. The hospital's reputation and good quality services have been a major attraction to different groups of customers. In terms of referral within and outside, the relationships with various groups of customers are judged to be very positive. The patients show preference and return to the same consultant, which is seen as a good sign of customer loyalty. Results of free camps in and around the town have been very successful also. Overall, this case hospital with more than 750 MBNQA points (out of 1000) is judged to be performing at golden level.

Case Study Inferences

The business orientation and healthcare focus have been integrated well in the hospital. Presently, there is a strong management commitment for enhancing quality of healthcare services and an intention to use quality as a competitive strategy (e.g., ISO certification and continuous improvement). Huge investments in the area of high technology and physical infrastructure artefacts indicate the healthcare leadership's focus on technical as well as service aspects of care. Areas of strategic planning, human resource training and development, standardizing healthcare processes and customer focus were strength areas of the hospital. Though a number of quality-based documentation and process standardization are initiated, measurement of data and data-driven improvement strategies need to be further improved. For instance, data and information on cost effectiveness, procedural appropriateness and risk management were not developed completely and explicitly shared with the researcher. Though Baldrige criteria allowed quality performance evaluation in all areas, the areas of administrative practices for streamlining patient/healthcare processes and legal procedures could not be directly explored in-depth. Also, the developing quality and service culture deserve to be seen as an independent criterion to further establish appropriate attitudes toward evidence-based quality practices among various staff. Therefore, it was found and validated by the managers of the hospital that servicescapes, service culture and administrative system be included as separate factors. This case study lends support to the appropriateness of the constructs selected from literature as critical to ensuring TQS in a hospital in this research work. The items of Baldrige healthcare criterion of organizational performance results are found to be very extensive and the hospital did not directly reveal data on a number of result areas. The managers identified the following key result areas as crucial: reputation of the hospital, patient care results, profitability, staff performance and success of new services.

The above case study provided support that the 13 quality constructs framework is appropriate in the Indian context. In order to further validate and select appropriate items (based on QM best practices) under each construct which would adequately measure the level of TQS in hospitals, an in-depth analysis of the hospital's best practices was carried out. The next section provides the details of the study.

Study Two

Qualitative Analysis of QM Practices in Indian Hospitals

The QM practices and their effectiveness are not published extensively as yet in the Indian context. In order to validate the contents of the 13 TQS constructs identified from literature analysis (presented in the previous chapter), it was decided to first understand and analyse if 'quality' was indeed considered as key to success of hospitals and second, to analyse quality management practices among reputed hospitals. The present paper details the content validation of the 13 TQS constructs through qualitative analysis of inputs from hospital managers.

Methodology

This study is exploratory in nature and content analysis of inputs from hospital managers was undertaken. A survey questionnaire containing different questions on hospital profile, technologies adopted, challenges faced, organization vision, mission and core values, quality policy, quality practices and barriers to effectively implement quality management in hospitals were developed (Appendix A). The questions and the checklist were selected so as to elicit relevant answers with a focus on 'quality practices' in hospitals. In addition, 25 senior hospital managers participated in in-depth interviews which gathered data on key success factor for hospitals, quality management practices and specific TQM-principle-based techniques that the organizations are using. Hospitals with more than 100 beds were chosen for the study as large hospitals have quality management practices/systems in place. In all, managers from 38 hospitals participated in the study and the data analysis is presented in the next section.

Results and Analysis

In general, the hospital population composed of multi-speciality/super-speciality acute care hospitals in India located across the north, south, east and west regions. Most of the hospitals included in this study are located in metro cities and only some are in towns or smaller cities. The hospitals have high reputation and hence considered to be providing high quality services (by virtue of being listed as major hospitals in yellow pages). The above criteria of hospital selection allowed for making generalizations on quality management criteria as they represent best practices in the industry and hence appropriate for validating quality performance factors. The data were analysed under the following sections, namely, challenges faced by hospitals, key success factor for hospitals and content analysis of quality management practices.

Challenges Faced by Hospitals

Based on the inputs of managers, the challenges can be classified under five major categories, namely:

1. *Competition among hospitals:* It was found to be true for almost all hospitals irrespective of the type of hospital namely corporate, trust-run, private or medical college hospital. Pricing, quality of services and specialists, use of technology

and ability to provide a stimulating working environment as well as benefits for staff were seen as important.

2. *Disease trends/epidemiology and disease management:* It was specifically mentioned that the challenges are to find specialists, e.g., oncologists for hospitals given the fact that prevalence of cancer in India is increasing. Disease management of life style diseases such as asthma, diabetes, kidney and heart as well as stress-related diseases were reported to be very challenging owing to their chronic nature.
3. *Providing services with cost effectiveness:* Opening up of departments in new specialty areas calls for huge investments, and the management is facing cost escalations. Resource allocation for new projects, costs of man power and technology along with increasing customer demands for better care are tipping the balance between costs and earnings. Achieving high volumes and high earnings is not easy in the sector. Thus, in the context of decreasing patient share (market share) and profits, cost effectiveness of expensive medical technologies were major concerns for hospital managers. Increasing use of technology in healthcare is a key factor in increasing cost of production of services.
4. *People focus and human resource management:* Another important area of concern for the hospital was manpower recruitment, training and retention especially retention of the nursing staff. Physician involvement and their almost unquestioned autonomy is another area of challenge for hospital managers especially while implementing newer management methods such as TQM.
5. *Changing trends in healthcare sector:* The growth of health-insurance sector is reportedly leading to increased documentation and man power training. In addition, demands by various customer groups for better services and value for money are seen as a threat in a sector which was predominantly provider-centric. Professional management and marketing of services once not so common in the industry are currently considered as crucial for survival in a competitive industry. The evolution of NABH standards is another change in the Indian healthcare sector. Some

hospital managers mentioned that the implementation of organization-wide TQM is a big challenge for hospital managers. The managers expressed that 'quality is an imperative', hospitals have to implement organization-wide quality management tools and techniques in order to excel. The competition in the sector is ever increasing and 'achieving excellence' cannot be ignored.

Key Success Factors for Hospitals

Table 7.2 shows the content analysis of the key success factor for hospitals as reported by the managers. The majority of hospitals mentioned 'quality' as a key success factor for hospitals. Most often quality of professionals and medical technology is reported to be very important for success. This research was carried out in 'reputed hospitals', which is based on customer perception as well as performance and the managers of those hospitals repeatedly reiterated that 'quality is critical to success'. Thus, they are congruent in nature.

Table 7.2

Key Success Factors for Hospitals

Key Success Factors	*Number of Hospitals**	*Specific Contents that Highlight the Factor (Survey/Interviews)*
Quality of Medical Care and Services	20 hospitals specifically mentioned 'quality' as a major success factor.	1. Quality of Medical Professionals 2. Quality of Medical Care and Services 3. Human Care
Medical Technology and Procedures	14 hospitals attributed the success to advanced technologies; 8 hospitals mentioned specialty and super-specialty care as key to their hospital's success.	1. Medical procedures and use of technologies including state-of-the-art technology. 2. Specific care facilities such as round-the-clock emergency, trauma care, laboratory services, total cancer/heart care, focused care areas such as ophthalmic, orthopedic, neurological care, etc.

Cont'd...

Cont'd...

Staffing	12 hospitals attributed the success to excellent staff.	1. Dedicated nursing staff 2. Excellent consultants/doctors 3. Personal involvement and passion 4. Team effort
Access and Affordability	6 hospitals	1. Affordability of specialized services 2. Ability to cater to a specific poverty-ridden geographical region the hospital is located in
Other Factors	One hospital each mentioned the reasons listed in the next column.	1. Brand image 2. Medical research 3. Corporate tie-ups 4. Insurance

*There were multiple responses and therefore the numbers do not add to the total number of hospitals (38) in the study.

Content Analysis of Quality Management Practices

All hospitals included in the study are formally carrying out some form of quality management programmes. They are using a range of quality practices which incorporate the principles of TQM. Cost efficiency and effectiveness is recognized to be very important by most interviewed.

The study explored how leadership and management commitment is manifest in hospitals with special reference to quality management practices. Leadership vision, mission, and clearly articulated values in general, indicate the leadership and management commitment to provide quality services to patients. Figure 7.1 shows the percentage of hospitals which have shown commitment to quality and professional management

The vision statements of hospitals were analysed for content and themes. Expansion of network of hospitals, excelling in all medical specialties, achieving patient satisfaction and providing high quality medical care with warm and professional service were the major themes in the vision statements of hospitals. The main theme of the mission statements was to provide ethical and quality care to all. Managers often referred to words such as 'world-class', 'international standards' and 'achieving excellence' while describing vision and mission.

Figure 7.1

Leadership and Management Commitment

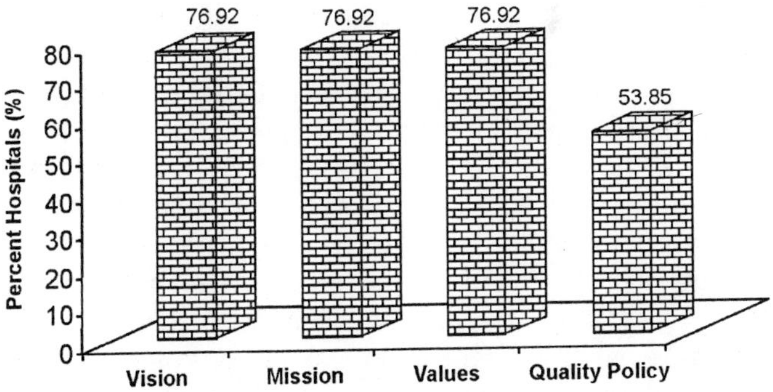

'Quality' appeared in vision, mission and value statements repeatedly; 'quality at all levels' is another value mentioned as important. Among the most important values mentioned in the survey are: Quality, Compassion, Integrity, Technical Excellence, Respect, Enthusiasm, Discipline, Customer Satisfaction, Equality, Honesty, Openness, Commitment and Hard Work. Quality policy was developed in only 53.85 per cent of the hospitals in the study. A total of 15 hospitals in the study have obtained ISO certification and five hospitals have Quality Assurance Departments. An important point to note: since the completion of this study, NABH compliance and certification is an important development in the Indian hospital sector.

Figure 7.2 shows that majority of the hospitals use more than one form of quality management methods. Further, it can be seen that Medical Audit (including medical records check) is the most common quality management procedure implemented in hospitals. Many hospitals also carry out customer and employee satisfaction surveys, the former being more frequently used than the latter. Benchmarking and 360 degree appraisal are the least frequently reported practices presently, but one respondent said that with increasing levels of awareness and information disclosure, such methods would be more frequently used in the future.

In addition to the checklist, respondents were requested to comment on the methods used for quality management in their respective hospitals. The following major points emerged from such qualitative information: Monitoring of hospital-acquired infection rates, mortality rates and morbidity rates are used to monitor the quality of care. The respondents said that process improvement was very important in achieving total quality. Such practices include standard process manuals/protocols for all departments and standard operating procedures (SOPs) for key processes as well as support services. Laboratories of 12 hospitals in the study are enrolled in external quality assurance and accreditation process by the National Accreditation Board for Laboratories (NABL). Training in quality, customer satisfaction surveys, periodic peer reviews and weekly appraisal through clinical society meetings are some of the other QM programmes carried out by the hospitals surveyed. Tools such as histograms, charts/tables, brainstorming techniques, data analysis and cause – effect diagram are used by respondent hospitals for data analysis in various departments/units. This survey clearly indicates that these large hospitals are implementing quality management and formalizing the practices.

Figure 7.2

QM Practices in Hospitals Surveyed

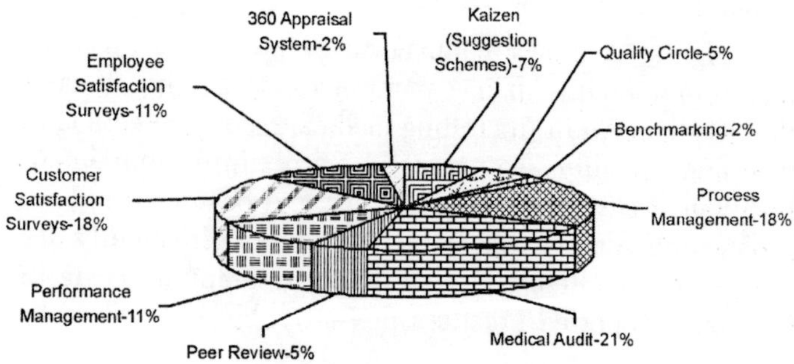

Responding to an open-ended question on additional inputs on 'quality' of healthcare services, the managers reported that hospital ambience, cleanliness and friendly atmosphere aspects important for patients, their families as well as for the staff. Staff training and professional management were also noted as crucial for enhancing efficiency and acquiring new knowledge.

Table 7.3 shows the detailed content analysis of quality management practices among Indian hospitals. This analysis clearly confirmed that the 13-construct TQS framework for hospitals is appropriate and useful.

Table 7.3

Detailed Analysis of Quality Management Practices among Indian Hospitals

Construct	*Quality Management Practices*	*Challenges*
Leadership and Management Commitment	• Communicating mission statement and quality policy through various channels such as meetings, displaying at various places, trainings, etc.	• Some managers reported that lack of leadership and management commitment as a major barrier for organization-wide TQM implementation.
	• Form core committees, open forums and proactive planning for ensuring quality practices.	
	• Allocate resources for quality management programmes.	
Strategic Planning	• Strategic partnerships with insurance companies, corporate contracts for providing services (e.g., Executive Health Check service package).	• It was noted that strategic planning was not carried out very systematically in the Indian hospital sector till recently.
	• Expansion of services based on analysis of data on external and internal environments in some hospitals.	

Cont'd...

Cont'd...

Human Resource Management and Development	• Enhanced training programmes for all level staff (e.g., from house-keeping, security to executives).	• Not all hospitals have job specifications and requirements formally written for all jobs.
	• Internal Quality Audits for HR (especially in ISO certified hospitals).	• Staff retention continues to be high especially among nurses (e.g., some managers said that the attrition rates are as high as 40%).
	• Continuing Medical/Nursing Education Programmes, sabbatical leave, training abroad used for Continuous Learning.	• One expert from a highly reputed medical college hospital said that employee training needs and actual training is still a 'token gesture' and lots need to be done.
	• Hospitals are addressing employee motivation and satisfaction more rigorously (e.g., rotation of HOD's in a department, career development, etc.)	• Physician autonomy and consultant model (vs. employing physicians) is challenging.
	• Compensation, support programmes, environmental-health-safety plans family support programmes, promotions.	
Healthcare Services-Design and Improvement	• Patient needs and requirements are considered for designing the services.	• Cost effectiveness of procedures.
	• A number of evaluation methods (especially performance indicators such as hospital infection rates, mortality and morbidity rates, clinical case discussion outputs)	• Procedural appropriateness based on data is very limited.

Cont'd...

Cont'd...

	• ICD and ICMR disease coding are used for streamlining the disease management. One hospital reported the use of DRG system.	• Physicians' unquestioned autonomy and use of traditional techniques makes redesigning of processes difficult.
	• Specific indicators for assessing disease management do not exist.	•
Process Management	• Many hospitals have identified core and support process.	• Ethical issues not strongly addressed (e.g., ethical committees not very common especially for professional and patient care related activities but may be found.
	• Standard operating procedures, departmental/clinical/nursing protocols, work instructions and procedure manuals have helped reduce variations in services.	• Not all hospitals in the study have SOPs for all departments.
	• Integration and streamlining of the various services.	
	• Measurement of processes and results need to be addressed.	
Servicescapes	• Hospital ambience and physical infrastructure being constantly improvised.	• Presently, a lot of investments are made to improve 'hotel like' services.
	• Cleanliness, hygiene and comfort for patients and employees are taken care of.	
	• Sign boards, ease of moving patients, stretchers, wheelchairs, paid due attention.	
	• Hotel like services improved with coffee shops, appealing front desks, attractive lounges, improved layouts, flower/book store, parking facilities, etc.	

Cont'd...

Cont'd...

Service Culture	• Friendly staff, a number of hospital representatives to help patients and families while being serviced. • Social work departments to assist patients with understanding treatment plans/procedures, payment options, etc. • Training staff in service culture, team work, helping nature and quality interactions.	• Establishing quality culture and team work needs to be strengthened.
Administrative System	• Integrating administrative and clinical processes. • Payments, billing, collection, claims and interdepartmental coordination given special attention. • Feedback from staff and patients/families on administrative procedures incorporated to improve services. • Regulatory mechanisms, forming committees for quality assurance set up. • ISO certification, accreditation by, National Board of Examination, hospital registration procedures, etc. are rigorously carried out. • Documentation and follow up of medico-legal cases streamlined in many hospitals.	• Coordinating various clinical and non-clinical processes in hospitals is reported to be lacking.

Cont'd...

Cont'd...

Measurement, Information and Analysis	• TQM practices such as Kaizen (suggestion schemes), quality circle, root cause analysis and benchmarking implemented in some hospitals.	• Data for benchmarking are not extensively available for Indian hospitals, published data for US hospitals are used as benchmarks in many instances, for example, hospital acquired-infection rates.
	• Data-driven tools and techniques implemented in cardiac surgeries, ICUs, OT/equipment utilization etc. to improve quality.	• Information technology based hospital information system are still being developed in most hospitals.
	• Data analysis and measurement of indicators such as post-operative infection rates, hospital-acquired infection rates, ventilator-pneumonia days, etc. are utilized to monitor the quality of care.	
	• Utilization rates, lab turn-around-time, medical record retrieval.	
	• Medical records check and quality of documentation done regularly.	
Supplier Quality Management	• Pharmacy supplies and just-in-inventory are implemented.	• Making 'quality' the most important criteria for vendor selection.
	• Quality checks on products and supplies well established in many hospitals.	
	• Annual Maintenance Contract for medical and other equipments.	
	• Vendor evaluation and raw material analysis for quality and costs carried out to ensure quality at reasonable costs.	

Cont'd...

Cont'd...

	• Long-term relationships with vendors established.	
Customer Focus and Satisfaction	• Customer satisfaction surveys are conducted on a regular basis. Developing a customer satisfaction index. • Motto of some hospitals 'Customer is the King' and 'Comfort to family'. • Handle grievances in a systematic manner. • Provide complaint boxes for customers to provide feedback on services. Some hospitals have published 'Bill of Rights for Patients'.	• Improving the validity of customer satisfaction surveys needs to be researched.
Key Results	• Profits, cost per procedures, bed occupancy, average length of stay are measured. • Reputation of the hospital, employee performance considered important indicators of overall organizational performance. • Number of in-patients and out-patients regularly monitored.	• Only rarely formal performance measurement techniques such as Balanced Score Card are used.
Social Responsibility	• Discounts to poor patients, free clinics in adopted villages, health camps to address issues of affordability. • One cancer hospital reported that treatment is not denied for lack of payments and a number of help is sought for patients.	• Increasing cost of medical care and use of high technology is affecting affordability factors. • Difficult to balance social equity issues with profit orientation given the high costs of technical care.

Cont'd...

Cont'd...

	• Corporate citizenship and community involvement regarded important. Unique programmes run by some hospitals in improving community awareness (e.g., health quiz for school students). • Telemedicine to improve accessibility to remote/rural people by some hospitals. • Improving environmental pollution through safe disposal of hospital wastes. Most hospitals follow Government of India Gazette Guidelines for hospital waste management.

Barriers to Implementation of Quality Management

A number of barriers were identified in the successful implementation of quality management by managers in the study. They are:

- Lack of top management commitment and resources;
- Staff resistance to change;
- Balancing between physicians' (consultants') autonomy and quality systems/processes;
- Diversity of working patterns and protocols;
- Apathy of the government sector;
- Lack of appropriate regulatory mechanisms (and their implementation) for Indian hospitals;
- Pharmaceutical competition which interferes with ethical practices;
- Lack of establishment of proper responsibility-accountability in case of problems;
- Hospitals continue to be highly centralized in authority relations is noted as a major barrier;
- Some managers opined that 'More means better', and that physicians and hospitals with time and facilities tend to do more tests, procedures, and use more advanced technology;

- Other managers reported that patients consider low price as a signal of poor quality and price sensitivity of patients is not always linear. However, pricing of services is still a major area contention in the sector;
- It was found that added features, 'hotel like' services have brought early successes in quality improvements (particularly based on perceptions of customers) but has pushed the costs of providing care. There should be incentives for healthcare professionals to improve health rather than increase the use of medical procedures is what a manager noted;
- Some feared that without real measure of outcomes, state-of-the-art facilities become focus of healthcare competition and not necessarily appropriateness of medical procedures and outcomes;
- Documentation and patterns of unusual rate of use of certain procedures (e.g., C-section deliveries or number of hysterectomies with severity adjusted rates) are not rigorously carried out by many hospitals; and
- Some managers complained about ISO certification being flaunted by a few hospitals and that no real change was perceptible.

These barriers along with challenges identified in Table 7.2 indicate that TQS implementation in India is rather in the initial phases. Evidence-based clinical and non-clinical practices have to be further improved.

Conclusions

The healthcare managers consider 'quality' as a very important competitive strategy in a fast growing industry. Quality management practices vary but basic principles of TQM such as customer orientation, improvement of technical quality based measurement and evidence is increasingly seen as important. A number of barriers and challenges have to be overcome in order to implement TQM successfully. Most hospital managers in the study reported that they are aligning resources, training employees and implementing programmes in order to achieve high quality.

The 13 TQS factors chosen through literature review analysis namely, Leadership and Management Commitment, Strategic

Planning, Administrative System, Supplier Quality Management, Process Management, Human Resource Management and Development, Healthcare Service Design and Improvement, Servicescapes, Service Culture, Measurement, Information and Analysis are systems, Customer Focus and Satisfaction, Key Results and Social Responsibility are found appropriate for implementing organization-wide quality management. A field study for assessing the reliability and validity of the proposed 13 TQS constructs for hospitals is judged to be highly relevant. Assessing the reliability would be best achieved using the internal consistency method (Cronbach's alpha) as it requires only one administration in a field study. Factor analysis can be carried out for validation of TQS constructs. Bivariate correlations between the TQS constructs based on the ratings on implementation levels of various quality constructs in hospitals in comparison to industry best practice would throw light on their relative importance.

Summary

This chapter presented the two empirical research studies for content validation of TQS constructs: one, quality performance measurement of a case hospital using MBNQA healthcare criteria and two, qualitative analysis of survey of Quality Management practices among Indian hospitals. Quality management practices based on TQM principles are becoming more prevalent in the Indian context and evolving rapidly in major hospitals. Customer orientation, hospital performance as a healthcare provider and a business enterprise, achieving high level of technical quality of care and cost effectiveness are becoming important in the hospital sector. The studies provided support to the appropriateness of the 13-construct TQS framework of this research and proved useful in improvising the measuring instrument for TQS. Reliability and validity testing of the 13 TQS constructs by field survey methodology would provide support and evidence to the usefulness of the framework. Further, refinement of the critical dimensions grouped under each quality construct would be useful as a quality measurement tool as well for implementation of organization-wide quality.

8

Empirical Investigation of TQS

Healthcare organizations especially hospitals are facing unparalleled challenges as many struggle to find ways to reduce costs while improving quality and productivity. Recent years have witnessed an increased interest in the TQM philosophy within healthcare organizations. It is being viewed as a means of increasing efficiency and improving the quality of care delivered. It is important for healthcare organizations to measure how they are performing on quality. However, traditional methods are proving inadequate given the complexity of activities, behaviours and procedures along with specialized knowledge that goes into producing high quality services. After a thorough examination of the literature, it was identified that a 13-construct structure would sufficiently measure the quality of healthcare services. Preliminary studies verified the criticality of the constructs and further empirical study was planned to test the reliability and validity of the constructs. This chapter focuses on the 'Designing of the TQS Measuring Instrument' and 'Empirical Validation of the TQS Framework'.

The overall research approach of this study consisted of the following phases:

1. *Identification, selection and explanation of TQS constructs:* Theoretical constructs of TQS are identified and selected based upon literature review and expert inputs – their analysis and synthesis (Chapters 2–6). The literature in quality management, organizational behaviour, general management theories and

healthcare quality management was thoroughly searched. Explanation of the TQS constructs is given in Appendix D.

2. *Designing TQS measuring instrument:* The measuring instrument should include items that would cover the entire range of TQS constructs with necessary scales for measurement of quality performance. Here again, research from empirical, practitioner and theoretical works of quality management as well as industry expert inputs provided a basis for the selection of measurement items. The items so selected were grouped under appropriate quality constructs identified from the literature. A questionnaire was developed to test and validate the TQS constructs. Questionnaire survey method has been acknowledged as an efficient tool for assessing the perceptions and experiences of a range of TQM practitioners from the industry. Survey questionnaire on quality measures is given in Appendix B.
3. *Content validation of TQS constructs:* Content validity of TQS constructs was verified by two expert survey studies. One study was an in-depth case (hospital) analysis using MBNQA Healthcare Criteria and second was a qualitative analysis of current practices in major hospitals using checklists, surveys and interviews. This was discussed in Chapter 7.
4. *TQS construct validation:* The TQS measuring instrument was tested using cross-sectional survey of hospital managers. Ratings of the items by the hospital managers formed the primary data and the ratings would be indicating the level of implementation of quality management behaviours, actions, and strategies under each TQS construct. Applying appropriate statistical methodologies, reliability and validity of the TQS constructs are determined. The present chapter, Chapter 8, discusses the main research study and analysis.
5. *Proposing an integrative TQS framework for hospitals:* Overall ratings of quality performance by hospital managers on various quality dimensions were compared to practices in the industry and interactions (correlations) between various TQS constructs were examined. Since the quality management strategies, actions and behaviours are interactive in nature and have to be applied holistically for achieving total quality, an integrated TQS framework for hospitals is proposed. This is presented in Chapter 9.

Research Methodology: Questionnaire, Sampling and Analysis Techniques

The literature review and analysis helped develop a 13-construct framework for TQS for hospitals. Two qualitative studies namely a case study on quality performance measurement based on MBNQA criteria and multi-hospital quality practices survey confirmed the appropriateness of the 13-construct framework (see Appendix A). The measurement model for this framework was developed in the form of a questionnaire. The constructs cannot be measured directly and can be operationalized using a scale or a set of items. Each scale was based on a thorough review and understanding of the literature, specifically healthcare quality literature, expert guidance and inputs from healthcare managers. The set of items most relevant to the construct being measured were selected from the literature on TQM (Chapter 6: Table 6.5) in which the item list was given. Majority of the items are traceable to the Baldrige Health Care Criteria (Meyer and Collier, 2001) and Kunst and Lemmink (2000). Items on the construct servicescapes, service culture and social responsibility are traceable to the holistic model for TQS as validated by Sureshchandar et al. (2001a, b) and supplier quality management to the instrument developed by Saraph et al. (1989), Ahire et al. (1996) and Meyer and Collier (2001). Items for the administrative system were identified from the studies by Lin and Clousing, 1995; Mohanty et al., 1996; Aggarwal and Zairi, 1997; Bharat et al., 1999; and Meyer and Collier, 2001 (MBNQA). The number of items (questions) was determined by ensuring that the content of the dimensions is adequately addressed. A number of points were noted down about quality management practices in hospitals to ensure that the items framed were appropriate for representing the respective scale/construct.

It was clearly noted that it was neither important nor feasible to include items that prescribe to particular methodologies or practices (as hospitals do not conform to the use of any one particular method) but that they should focus on whether the relevant management and quality issues are addressed thoroughly.

For instance, the scale item on the dimension on Measurement, Information and Analysis, an item reads: "We use a number of statistical tools to analyse data in a number of areas", it does not prescribe whether specific methods such Run Charts or Histograms should be used. To improve comprehension and reduce ambiguities, experts from the field suggested modifications on the items. One of the most important modifications was to provide examples of methods or a group of techniques that may be actually practiced. For example, the scale item on the dimension on Healthcare Service Design and Improvement, an item reads: "Our hospital uses a number of patient health care results/indicators for evaluation of service (mortality/morbidity rates, patient length of stay, disease-specific mortality rates, etc.)". Since the industry's best practice and indicators of performance are not uniform, the experts suggested that including some examples would provide cues and thereby ensure uniformity in comprehension of questions. Three revisions of questionnaire development were carried out after the initial selection of items. Experts from hospital management and TQM experts reviewed the questions. After, eliminating and/or reclassifying certain items, the remaining items were administered to a total of six hospital and healthcare managers including hospital administrators, medical superintendents and heads of the departments. During these pretest interviews, the managers commented on the clarity of specific items, critiqued their ease of comprehension and suggested changes to improve their wording. Following this, 118 measurement items grouped into 13 factors were retained (Appendix B).

Following similar studies (e.g., Saraph et al., 1989; Zhang et al., 2000) a five-point Likert-type equal interval scale was employed for scoring responses. Managers had to indicate the degree or extent of practice of each item by their hospital utilizing a scale anchor of 1=Not at all; 2=Occasionally; 3=Somewhat; 4=Frequently; 5=Always for all constructs except for Key Results the scale anchor was 1=Very Low; 2=Low; 3=Medium; 4=High and 5=Very High.

A typical example is shown here:

'Our focus on patients originates from within management'.

1	2	3	4	5

Sampling Plan

A *multi-stage sampling technique* was used in selecting the respondents for the empirical research. A *sampling frame of 65 major hospitals* was constructed from a list of major hospitals in India from yellow pages of telephone directory (Bangalore Medical Directory, 2005) and professional associations. Fifty were listed as major hospitals and another 15 were included based on expert recommendations (based on the following criteria: quality of care, range/size of service operation and reputation) in order to obtain a larger population frame. In general, the hospital population composed of multi-speciality/super-speciality acute care hospitals in India located across the north, south, east and west regions.

The following reasons determined the criteria for hospital selection:

1. Multi-speciality care hospitals provide a wide variety of medical services and are complex organizations and hence the evaluation of their practices provides a logical basis for establishing and validating quality performance factors, which is the main objective of this research.
2. Hospitals with more than 100 beds were chosen for the study as large hospitals have quality management practices/systems in place. This was further strengthened by the fact that most of hospitals in the population frame are listed as a major hospital and therefore each hospital has high reputation and is providing high quality care.

The study is to be conducted at the facility level with Senior Manager as a sampling unit. At the hospital level, more than one respondent group was included for the study, namely, top-and middle-level managers referred to as Senior Managers. Research has shown that this type of respondent selection provides a true picture of implementation level as top management is usually involved in planning and mid-level managers are actively involved in implementation (Counte and Meurer, 2001; Sureshchandar et al., 2001b).

Scale Refinement and Validation

Conventionally, studies in organizational behaviour and marketing research utilize Exploratory Factor Analysis for factor identification and refinement. Similar approach has been found useful in research on critical factors for TQM (e.g., Saraph et al., 1989; Black and Porter, 1996). Such an approach to scale refinement consists of the following steps (Ahire et al., 1996):

- Theoretical and conceptual background in a particular domain is clearly deciphered through an extensive literature review and a subsequently critical dimension of the construct that is intended to be measured is identified.
- Design and develop a survey instrument to measure those constructs by carefully selecting the items to measure each scale. This would also involve pre-testing of the instrument either objectively or subjectively by experts in the field for content validity. Finally, the measurement instrument is revised and refined.
- A field study (survey method) is carried out to test the instrument.
- Data analysis is performed using an exploratory factor analysis (often with varimax rotation) on item responses to extract latent factors according to item-factor loadings. EFA seeks to uncover the underlying structure of a relatively large set of variables. The researcher's á priori assumption is that any indicator may be associated with any factor. There is no prior theory and one uses factor loadings to intuit the factor structure of the data.
- Refining the scales using Cronbach's scale reliability coefficient alpha.

All the above steps have been carried out in the present research and for the data analysis, the Confirmatory Factor Analysis (CFA) is opted. Research in TQM construct validation has used such an approach, notably by Ahire et al. (1996) and

Sureshchandar et al. (2001b). Also, there is an increasing acceptance of CFA in organizational and marketing research as noted by Ahire et al. (1996). Since the present research developed the constructs on sound theoretical and empirical research in the area of healthcare as well as expert inputs, the researcher chose to adopt the factor analysis using a confirmatory method. A minimum requirement of CFA is that one hypothesizes beforehand the number of factors in the model, usually the researcher will also posit expectations about which variables will load on which factors. Then, the researcher seeks to determine, for instance, if the measures created to represent a latent variable really belong together. The CFA can be accomplished through any general-purpose statistical package that supports factor analysis. Scale reliability was tested for internal consistency which can be estimated using a reliability coefficient of Crocnbach's alpha (α).

Correlations between Constructs

The TQS programmes in professional service organizations, such as hospitals need to use both profession-specific and modern organizational quality methods to develop personnel and organization in an integrated way. Study of relationships between various constructs was carried out by analysing correlations by the following researchers: Ahire et al. (1996), Ang et al. (2000), Zhang et al. (2000) and Sureshchandar et al. (2001b). This study particularly would follow the method used by Zhang et al. (2000), which considered the perceptual ratings based on comparison of quality performance of an organization to industry best practice. The relationships among 13-construct TQS framework would be tested using bivariate correlation (Pearson's) based on the ratings of quality performance on each construct in comparison to the industry best practice by quality experts from major hospitals. Positive correlations would indicate that TQS constructs are interrelated and that the quality management efforts should be applied in a holistic manner rather than piecemeal.

Having arrived at a 13-construct TQS framework for hospitals and selected an appropriate methodology to validate model, the following hypothesis is defined for the study:

TQS framework for hospitals is a 13-construct structure consisting of the following constructs only: Leadership and Management Commitment; Strategic Planning; Human Resource Management and Development; Healthcare Service Design and Improvement; Process Management; Service Culture; Servicescapes; Administrative System; Measurement, Information and Analysis; Supplier Quality Management; Customer Focus & Satisfaction; Key Results; and Social Responsibility.

Sample Characteristics

The survey was conducted in the year 2005 on selected healthcare organizations and it focused on the extent and nature of quality management in these organizations in the Indian context. It is an investigation of quality management implementation in hospitals, both small and large that provide a wide variety of healthcare services. The cross-sectional survey method was applied because of its effectiveness as a tool for gathering a 'snapshot' of information about the subject under research. Following a case study and an exploratory study of expert inputs, a personalized self-completion questionnaire was administered with detailed explanation of the nature and purpose of the research. The questionnaire was designed so as to elicit information on the key issues identified within the literature review and was as a result divided into 13 sections containing questions relating to each construct of TQS (Appendix B).

This study is conducted at the facility level with Senior Manager as a sampling element. Once the necessary permission was obtained from the hospital administration, the Senior Managers were contacted and given the questionnaire personally, through mail or email.

Of the 65-hospital population frame, it was possible to contact at least one Senior Manager (such as CEO or Medical Director or Chief Hospital Administrator) in 43 hospitals. A total of 425 Senior Managers were administered the questionnaires, out of which nearly about a 100 were administered personally and the rest by mail. Out of the 43 hospitals, 29 hospitals responded and the managers sent back the filled questionnaires. Follow up was carried out through telephone calls and emails to increase the response rate. Eleven of the questionnaires were incompletely filled and therefore were not included for further analysis. Finally, a sample size of 146 was achieved. Overall, 44.62 per cent hospitals responded (29 out of 65) and there was 67.44 per cent, i.e., 29 out of 43 where personal contact was established with one or more Senior Managers. 34.35 per cent (146 out of 425) filled questionnaires were analysed. This high rate of return was possible because of the following reasons:

- Personal contact approach in the form of initial contact for prior consent to participate contributed to the successful questionnaire return rate.
- Follow up through emails, mail and phone calls was carried out to increase response rate.

A small number of missing data points in these 146 filled questionnaires were replaced with scale average scores However, it was in just 12 item responses, that is in a total of 17,228 (118 X 146) item responses and hence the data gaps are not significant. Sample size adequacy (146 in all) is judged to be satisfactory as the number of responses is more than the items in the measuring instrument (118 items under 13 constructs), a minimum requirement for sample size for statistical analysis purposes. Also, considering the difficulties faced such as reluctance/refusals to participate and time delays due to permissions from the hospitals, a sample size of 146 from reputed hospitals in the country is considered adequate.

Table 8.1 shows the distribution of respondents and the number of hospitals in the study sample by bed size categories (five groups). The maximum number of respondent hospitals is from hospitals under 500 beds. These hospitals are of national or regional repute by the fact that a majority of them is listed as major hospitals in India, many hospitals are quite popular and known for their quality of services. The respondent hospital list is given in the Appendix C in alphabetical order. In almost all hospitals, more than one Senior Manager participated in the study. In general, the number of responses per hospital increased with increasing size of the hospital (larger hospitals would correspondingly have more Senior Managers too). Overall, the sample size and the number of respondent hospitals are judged to represent the hospital population frame of the study quite well and hence the results from the study could be generalized for the hospital population under study.

Table 8.1

Distribution of Respondents (Senior Managers) Among Hospitals

Number of Beds	*Number of Hospitals*	*Number of Respondents*	*Range of Average Outpatients Per Day Among the Hospitals*
100–299	11	24	200–1200
300–499	10	62	150–700
500–699	1	4	280
700–899	4	5	250–1100
>900	3	51	600–1500
Total	**29**	**146**	

Table 8.2 further shows the hospital characteristics based on type of services provided, ownership of the hospitals, ISO certification for hospitals, turn over and growth rates. Majority of the hospitals have private ownership and three medical college hospitals also participated. In general, the sample of hospitals in the study provides a wide variety of services to a large number of patients. The categorization of multi or super-speciality care is based on the services the hospitals provide. The sample size and the type of organizations included in the study are judged to be sufficient for drawing conclusions about quality management practices. The hospitals in the sample (and population frame) truly represent the industry best practice, ones based on their reputation, customer base and listing as major hospitals.

Table 8.2 on respondent hospital characteristics also shows data on the average turn over in crores which is ₹ 77.27 crores for the year 2004–05 with a range of 8–225 crores. The data on turn over are just an indication of the level of operations of the hospitals in the study and since only 11 hospitals provided the data, no further attempt was made to analyse the level of business operations. The average annual growth rate reported was 36.25 per cent growth rate with a range of 10 to 80 per cent. A growth rate of 36.25 per cent is much higher than the industry average of 15 per cent growth reported in the country and it indicates the respondent hospitals are doing well. Again, the fact that the growth rate was disclosed by only eight hospitals implies that the value has to be interpreted carefully as it may not be the true representation of the growth rate of all the hospitals in the study. But, other factors such as the reputation, the listing as a major hospital and the number of outpatients (as well as in-patients treated) indicate that the hospitals are very successful. Table 8.2 gives the respondents' (Senior Managers') characteristics.

Table 8.2

Respondent Hospital Characteristics

Type of Services	*Multi/Super-Speciality (22)*	*Multi-Speciality (3)*	*Super-Speciality (4)*	
Ownership of Hospitals	Company Ltd. (15)	Trust Hospitals (11)	Medical College Hospital (Private 3; One Deemed University under UGC)	
ISO Certification	ISO 9001 (5)	ISO 9002 (5)	ISO 140001 (1)	Initiating ISO/JCI Certification (1)

Cont'd...

Cont'd...

Average Turnover in Crores of Rupees (2004–2005)	77.27* (only 11 hospitals disclosed the information)
Average Growth Rate (2004–2005)	36.25%* (only 8 hospitals disclosed the information)

* Number in parentheses indicates the number of hospitals under a particular category. The values indicate average turn over and growth rate for the hospitals surveyed.

Table 8.3

Respondent Characteristics (Total Number = 146)

Character	*Details*
Experience	• Average 13.80 years • Range 1 to 32 years
Background	• 89 were Medical (Clinician Managers) • 13 were from Nursing • 44 Managers (Non-clinician Managers)
Management Level	• 44.52% (65/146) were from Top Management
Position/Titles (Titles are typical examples, a wide variety of titles are generally followed)	• Top Management: Executive Director, Chief Executive Officer, Vice President, General Manager Operations, Senior Executive Health Care Services, Chief Hospital Administrator, Nursing Director, Head Medical Services, Dean/Principal Medical/Nursing College, Director Clinical Services, General Manager Customer Care, Vice President Human Resources • Mid-Level Management: Heads of the Departments (in some hospitals HODs formed a part of top management, so the distinction for some is not always clear cut), Hospital Administrators, Manager Health Care Services, Senior Consultant, Senior Scientific Officer, Public Relations Officer, Corporate Relations Officer, Associate Hospital Administrator, Medical Superintendents

Reliability Analysis

Table 8.4 reports the original sets of measurement associated with the 13 constructs and the reliability coefficient, the Cronbach's

Table 8.4

Internal Consistency Analysis Results for TQS Constructs (Reliability Analysis-Cronbach's Alpha)

Construct	*No. of Items**	*Item Means for Scale*	*Means of Inter Item Covariance*	*Means of Inter Item Correlation*	*Cronbach Alpha (α)*	*Standardized Item Alpha(α)*
Leadership and Management Commitment	9 (1–9)	3.9825	0.3094	0.3624	0.8366	0.8365
Strategic Planning	8 (10–17)	3.7517	0.3724	0.3905	0.8313	0.8367
Human Resource Management and Development	16 (18–33)	3.5509	0.5054	0.4137	0.9198	0.9186
Healthcare Service Design and Improvement	12 (34–45)	3.8322	0.4386	0.3954	0.8847	0.8870
Process Management	9 (46–54)	3.9962	0.5000	0.4675	0.8877	0.8877
Service Culture	5(55–59)	3.3959	0.6167	0.5540	0.8608	0.8613
Servicescapes	6 (60–65)	3.9863	0.4758	0.4634	0.8376	0.8383
Administrative System	7(66–73)	3.7483	0.5183	0.3990	0.8450	0.8416
Measurement, Information and Analysis	14 (74–87)	3.7074	0.6754	0.5264	0.9392	0.9396
Supplier Quality Management	6 (88–93)	3.9269	0.4265	0.4482	0.8286	0.8298
Customer Focus and Satisfaction	9 (94–102)	3.9277	0.5536	0.4988	0.9001	0.8996
Key Results	6 (103–108)	3.6062	0.1562	0.3445	0.7579	0.7592
Social Responsibility	10 (109–118)	3.9500	0.3874	0.3694	0.8516	0.8542
Overall Reliability	118 (1–118)	3.8174	0.3705	0.3414	0.9841	0.9839

*Numbers in parenthesis indicate the item numbers in serial order as it appears in the SPSS data file.

Note: None of the items are deleted at this stage, as alpha values are high for all constructs.

alpha (α) values for all the 13 scales. All statistical analysis was carried out using SPSS Version 11.5 software. Although, dropping some items from scales with lower correlation would improve some alpha values, no items were deleted to improve the alpha values (Table 8.4), which are high and meet the criterion of exceeding 0.7 for all the scales. Also, this was done in order to ensure the content validity of each measurement scale. The reliability analysis for all the constructs showed an α value of more than 0.82 except for the construct key results. Alpha value of 0.70 or above is considered to be the criterion for demonstrating internal consistency of established scales (Nunnaly, 1988). The range of α value from 0.7579 to 0.9392 indicates that some constructs are more reliable than the others.

Item Analysis

Item analysis was done, and mean and standard deviation were computed. Individual item averages indicated an overall high average which means that the implementation levels of many areas of quality management are quite high. Items in Human Resource Management and Development (HRM&D) showed the lowest means when compared to all other constructs which shows that HRM&D strategy implementation is perhaps lower. The following items under various constructs emerged as most important (based on highest mean among the items for each construct):

Construct	*Item with Highest Mean*
Leadership and Management Commitment	'Our senior executives focus on improving patient care'
Strategic Planning	'Our strategies address performance as both a healthcare provider and a business enterprise'
Human Resource Management and Development	'We derive employee hiring and development objectives from strategic objectives'
Healthcare Service Design and Improvement	'Procedures and possible outcomes are explained to patients so they know what to expect'

Cont'd...

Cont'd...

Process Management	'We obtain feedback on support services from patients and improve further'
Service Culture	'All the employees realize that the real purpose of their work is service to patients/customers'
Servicescapes	'The signboards, symbols, advertisements boards, pamphlets and other artefacts in the hospital are appealing to the customers'
Administrative System	'The legal aspects of care and other management/administrative procedures are streamlined and backed by data/appropriate documentation. (Such as medico-legal cases, employee complaints, disputes)'
Measurement, Information and Analysis	'Our information systems are standardized across departments (patient care, accounting, etc.)'
Supplier Quality Management	'Quality is our most important criterion for selecting suppliers than just price' and 'We provide clear specifications to suppliers'
Customer Focus and Satisfaction	'Customer focus and quality are driving forces behind day-to-day operations'
Key Results	'Reputation of the hospital'
Social Responsibility	'We address environmental health/pollution issues with appropriate measures (e.g., disposing biomedical/hazardous materials appropriately, training staff and other customers involved in disposal, etc.)'

Validity Analysis

The face and content validity analysis refers to goodness-of-fit of items within a scale. Face validity is qualitatively determined through the researcher's intuitive judgement during the process of identification and selection of constructs. Insights gained through literature analysis and expert inputs strengthen the face validity in this research. Content validity is established through the selection of constructs based on a comprehensive analysis and synthesis of literature review. The analysis also included specifics of healthcare criteria through different modes of research, namely conceptual, prescriptive, practitioner and empirical research. Based on such an analysis, the instrument was developed. Further, experts in the field of TQM and healthcare quality practitioners reviewed the items selected and found them valid. The results of qualitative research methods of case study and interviews of hospital managers at various stages help establish content validity.

Table 8.5

Kaiser-Meyer-Olkin (KMO) Measure of Sampling Adequacy for TQS Constructs

Construct	*No. of Items**	*Items deleted (by number)*	*KMO*
Leadership and Management Commitment	9 (1–9)	None	0.853
Strategic Planning	8 (10–17)	None	0.848
Human Resource Management and Development*	16 (18–33)	None	0.911
Healthcare Service Design and Improvement*	12 (34–45)	None	0.867
Process Management	9 (46–54)	None	0.866
Service Culture	5 (55–59)	None	0.788
Servicescapes	6 (60–65)	None	0.809
Administrative System*	7 (66–73)	None	0.812
Measurement, Information and Analysis*	14 (74–87)	None	0.912
Supplier Quality Management	6 (88–93)	None	0.815
Customer Focus and Satisfaction	9 (94–102)	None	0.895
Key Results	6 (103–108)	None	0.813
Social Responsibility	10 (109–118)	None	0.860

*Constructs 3, 4, 8 and 9 did not meet the unifactorial criteria and were split in factor analysis, the factor analysis and KMOs for split factors will be discussed later.

Factor Analysis

Factor analysis was carried out for 13 constructs used in the study for construct validity and scale unidimensionality. Prior to performing the factor analysis, the data matrix was examined to ensure that it had sufficient correlations to justify the application of factor analysis. One of the measures to quantify the degree of intercorrelations among the variables and the appropriateness of factor analysis is the Kaiser-Meyer-Olkin (KMO) measure of sampling adequacy. A small value of KMO means that each variable cannot be predicted or explained by the other variables without significant error; hence factor analysis may not be appropriate. As a guideline, KMO values in the 0.90s are considered as marvellous; 0.80s are meritorious; 0.70s are middling; 0.60s are mediocre; 0.50s are miserable and below 0.50s are unacceptable (Hair et al., 1995 cited in Ang et al., 2000, p. 57). Individual variables that have KMO values lower than 0.50 should be considered for exclusion. All constructs in the study showed higher values and that they could be taken up for factor analysis.

Factor loadings and data matrix is given in Table 8.6. We can infer that for the construct 'Leadership and Management Commitment', the first factor has an Eigen value of 3.935. Since this is greater than 1.0, it explains more variance than a single variable, in fact 3.935 times as much. The per cent of variance explained by this factor is 43.72 per cent. For the construct 'Social Responsibility', the first factor has an Eigen value of 4.368. It indicates that this factor explains more variance than a single variable, in fact 4.368 times as much. In general, the per cent of variance explained by the factors fell in the range of 43.506 (Key Results) to 64.399 (Social Responsibility).

Taking a closer look at the factor loadings of these nine constructs, majority of the individual items show loadings in the range of 0.6 and 0.8, which indicates the appropriateness of the items in the scale. Only six items have factor loadings below 0.6. It can be noted that statistically 0.3 and above is considered good enough. And also, it was of interest to see if the items had any specific explanatory power in the light of the results. These items in general showed lower item means than other items in their respective groups.

Using the CFA for the constructs, each construct was subjected to an individual Principal Component Analysis using SPSS programme's data reduction analysis (factor analysis). Scale unidimensionality was tested and confirmed for each scale using the data collected from 146 Senior Managers of 29 major hospitals. If each factor was valid as a construct, then its set of variables would form a single factor (unifactorial or unidimensional in nature). Carmines and Zeller (1979) guidelines as cited in Meyer and Collier (2001, pp. 411–12) were followed to determine the Factor Analysis statistics. The per cent of variance explained by the first principal component of each measurement scale was considered as important. One criterion is that the first component of each scale explains more than 40 per cent of the variance in the items. The second criterion is that the factor loadings for items should be greater than 0.30, in fact, this study considered items whose factor loadings are greater than 0.40. The two remaining criteria considered were: a large Eigen value for the first component and small, fairly equal Eigen values for subsequent components for subsequent components.

Unidimensionality measure is a must for constructs so that the items grouped together under each construct estimate single construct. In the present research, the constructs were pre-specified and hence were subjected to a tentative test of unidimensionality. Using the CFA for the constructs, each construct was subjected to an individual Principal Component Analysis using SPSS programme's data reduction analysis (factor analysis).

The factor matrix for the 13 constructs of TQS for hospitals is presented in Table 8.6. In this measure, each factor was assumed to be a separate construct. The results show that the driving systems of Leadership and Management Commitment System and Strategic Planning and the goals of TQS, namely, Customer Focus and Satisfaction, Key Results and Social Responsibility dimensions were unifactorial. Also, among the TQS enabling systems, the following constructs, namely, Process

Management, Service Culture, Servicescapes and Supplier Quality Management, all showed a clear scale unidimensionality. That is, nine constructs out of the 13 were clearly unidimensional in nature in the study and the four factors, namely, Human Resource Management and Development, Healthcare Service Design and Improvement, Administrative System, and Measurement, Information and Analysis split into two to three sub-factors. Table 8.6 also shows the data matrix for all the factors with number of factors under each construct, Eigen values, factor loadings and per cent variance explained by the factor. The factors that split were again subjected to similar kind of analysis to ensure reliability and validity. These factors were sent to a panel of experts independently for labelling the newly grouped items in order to ensure content validity and through a three-stage process using Delphi technique were labelled a suitable name. The details of factor analysis and labelling process are discussed in the following sections.

Analysis of Four Split Factors

This part presents the results and discussion of four constructs which did not fulfill the criteria of unidimensionality in factor analysis and split into two to three sub-factors. Empirical research studies have shown such splitting of factors after factor analysis and the decision by researchers to include them as separate factors are based on other statistics such as Eigen values, KMO values and per cent variance explained by the set of sub-factors (Saraph et al., 1989; Ang et al., 2000; Zhang et al., 2000). Since the aim of using quality-related information is to evaluate an organization's quality management practices and that the items were carefully selected to represent the scales chosen, the researchers argue that the factor split is not to be considered as crucial. In fact, interpretations should be based on the total view of research contents and sampling frame. Without such caution it is possible to overstate the statistical findings (Madu, 1998 cited in Zhang et al., 2000). The results warrant further research to evaluate the construct scales of the four split factors. One possibility is that this type of

Table 8.6

Results of Factor Analysis for 13 TQS Constructs

Constructs	*Number of Factors*	*Eigen Values*	*Factor Loadings*										
			Item 1	Item 2	Item 3	Item 4	Item 5	Item 6	Item 7	Item 8	Item 9	Item 10	% Of Variance
1. Leadership and Management Commitment	1	3.935	0.797 (1)*	0.665 (2)	0.635 (3)	0.65 1 (4)	0.590 (5)	0.693 (6)	0.698 (7)	0.541 (8)	0.659 (9)		43.722
2. Strategic Planning	1	3.767	0.724 (10)	0.669 (11)	0.663 (12)	0.581 (13)	0.592 (14)	0.811 (15)	0.709 (16)	0.713 (17)			47.087
3. Human Resource Management and Development	3	5.183 (Factor 1)	0.614 (20)	0.711 (21)	0.699 (22)	0.775 (26)	0.737 (27)	0.668 (29)	0.779 (30)	0.635 (31)	0.802 (32)	0.754 (33)	51.834
		2.379 (Factor 2)	0.686 (23)	0.859 (24)	0.785 (25)	0.745 (28)							59.471
		1.558 (Factor 3)	0.883 (18)	0.883 (19)									77.891
4. Healthcare Service Design and Improvement	2	3.892 (Factor 1)	0.742 (34)	0.753 (35)	0.828 (36)	0.726 (37)	0.744 (38)	0.742 (39)	0.677 (40)				55.605
		2.685 (Factor 2)	0.797 (41)	0.798 (42)	0.748 (43)	0.696 (44)	0.607 (45)						53.698
5. Process Management	1	4.777	0.779 (46)	0.715 (47)	0.794 (48)	0.787 (49)	0.734 (50)	0.617 (51)	0.738 (52)	0.770 (53)	0.594 (54)		53.078

Cont'd...

Cont'd...

6. Service Culture	1	3.220	0.772 (55)	0.773 (56)	0.807 (57)	0.802 (58)	0.856 (59)					64.399
7. Servicescapes	1	3.321	0.787 (60)	0.733 (61)	0.708 (62)	0.713 (63)	0.759 (64)	0.761 (65)				55.352
8. Administrative System	2	3.117 (Factor 1)	0.750 (66)	0.811 (67)	0.842 (68)	0.785 (69)	0.756 (70)					62.341
		1.831 (Factor 2)	0.386 (71)	0.449 (72)	0.442 (73)							61.025
9. Measurement, Information and Analysis	3	4.009 (Factor 1)	0.743 (76)	0.750 (80)	0.836 (81)	0.857 (82)	0.862 (86)	0.847 (87)				66.813
		3.428 (Factor 2)	0.788 (74)	0.826 (75)	0.808 (77)	0.846 (78)	0.869 (79)					68.557
		2.177 (Factor 3)	0.841 (83)	0.877 (84)	0.837 (85)							72.628
10. Supplier Quality Management	1	3.254	0.651 (88)	0.731 (89)	0.748 (90)	0.740 (91)	0.821 (92)	0.718 (93)				54.237
11. Customer Focus and Satisfaction	1	5.024	0.717 (94)	0.694 (95)	0.805 (96)	0.713 (97)	0.777 (98)	0.770 (99)	0.790 (100)	0.828 (101)	0.603 (102)		55.818
12. Key Results	1	2.730	0.672 (103)	0.655 (104)	0.678 (105)	0.632 (106)	0.644 (107)	0.758 (108)				45.506
13. Social Responsibility	1	4.368	0.592 (109)	0.623 (110)	0.701 (111)	0.734 (112)	0.567 (113)	0.600 (114)	0.711 (115)	0.563 (116)	0.757 (117)	0.722 (118)	43.682

* Numbers in parentheses indicate the item numbers as they appeared in the SPSS data file during the analysis.

research work using cross-sectional survey of hospitals for identification and validation of constructs for TQS is being conducted when the quality management practices are beginning to evolve in the Indian healthcare sector. Hence, the perceptions of criticality of practice may vary more in the Indian context than in other healthcare systems in which the TQS practices have reached a mature stage (for instance, the case of the US as seen in Meyer and Collier's 2001 study). However, the other statistical measures, namely Eigen values, per cent variance explained and measure of sampling adequacy indicate that the constructs and the items are properly selected and hence validate the criticality of the constructs in question. Though the factors have split, the original

Table 8.7
Labelling of Sub-factors

Construct	*Sub-factors*
Construct 3	**Sub factors – 3**
Human Resource Management and Development	1. Employee Well-being and Empowerment
	2. Training
	3. Human Resource Planning
Construct 4	**Sub factors – 2**
Healthcare Service Design and Improvement	1. Healthcare Service Design
	2. Healthcare Service Continuous Improvement
Construct 8	**Sub factors – 2**
Administrative System	1. General Administration
	2. Legal Administration
Construct 9	**Sub factors – 3**
Measurement, Information and Analysis	1. Information and Analysis
	2. Hospital Information System
	3. Performance Management

construct can be considered to consist of sub-factors. It can be argued from the analysis of theoretical and quality management practice literature that the items under the factors are closely related to the original construct rather than being seen as a separate construct. Four constructs split into more than one sub-factor and were further subjected to reliability and validity analysis (Appendix C).

The constructs were retained as originally constructed (with sub-factors) based on logical grouping of items and statistical analysis which indicated high Eigen values, factor loadings and per cent of variance in unrotated factor structure for all these factors. Using the Delphi expert consensus building technique, the sub-factors were labelled to ensure content validity. Table 8.7 shows the four constructs which split and the sub-factors under each of them.

Summary

This chapter presented the results and discussion of the testing and analysis of the TQS measuring instrument with 118 items grouped appropriately as 13 quality constructs. Face and Content validity was determined by literature review analysis and expert inputs. Applying the cross-sectional survey methodology, the instrument was administered to 146 Senior Managers of 29 major hospitals in India. The managers rated each item on a five-point Likert scale indicating the implementation level of Quality Management strategy in their respective hospitals. Statistical analysis was carried out for the data collected using SPSS Version 11.5. The analysis included Cronbach's alpha coefficient for reliability, descriptive statistics for items (mean and standard deviation), Kaiser – Meyer – Olkin (KMO) Measure of Sampling Adequacy and construct validity for unidimensionality using CFA with the help of Principal Component Analysis. All the items of the instrument were found to be highly reliable. Nine factors out of 13 were confirmed for unidimensionality and four factors were split into more than one sub-factor. The four factors were further subjected to reliability and validity analysis, and were retained as valid constructs with sub-factors. Using the Delphi expert consensus building technique, the sub-factors were labelled to ensure content validity. The development of the conceptual model based on relationships among the constructs is discussed in the next chapter.

9

Integrative Framework for Total Quality Service Management in Hospitals

Research on quality constructs for achieving Total Quality Service (TQS) in hospitals showed that total quality could be achieved by cperationalizing the 13 critical factors and QM strategies. The next question is obvious: "What is the relationship among the various constructs?" Establishing cause-effect is not easy when multiple factors are involved. However, the starting point is that of closely examining research literature in order to understand the relationships among the constructs.

Practitioners of Total Quality Service Management would have a keen interest in understanding how the TQS constructs are related. Understanding of such relationships would provide specific directions for implementation. The questions that arise are: What are the causal relationships of various constructs in achieving high quality? Will the manager be able to achieve high level outputs by applying QM strategies in a linear fashion? Do the constructs contribute equally to achievement of TQS, etc. At the first level, researchers develop a conceptual model based on the understood relationships among the constructs. Insights from literature analysis and expert inputs provide guidelines to researchers to develop a conceptual framework. The following section discusses the frameworks from literature. Later bivariate correlation among the 13 TQS constructs is studied. Finally, a conceptual 'Integrated TQS Management Model' is developed.

Total Quality Service Management Frameworks

Most quality awards include the criteria of Leadership, Strategy and Policy Planning, Resources, Information and Analysis, Customer Focus and Satisfaction, People Management, Process Management, Management of Suppliers/Partners, Performance and Business Results. The award criteria evolved over a period of time, e.g., MBNQA criteria and sub-criteria established since 1987 has shifted emphasis from quality assurance to process management to quality management and now to overall performance management in the USA. All the three award criteria are prescriptive in nature but only Deming Prize clearly indicates the tools, techniques and practices, and every factor is weighed equally for contributing to overall organizational progress. The Deming Prize is not based on an underlying framework linking concepts, activities, processes and results together with a causality relationship but provides a list of good quality oriented management practices. On the other hand, MBNQA and EQA attempt to model a causal relationship among different constituents of TQM. The causal relationships of MBNQA and EQA are given in Figures 9.1 and 9.2.

Figure: 9.1

Relationships among MBNQA Criteria (Source: NIST)

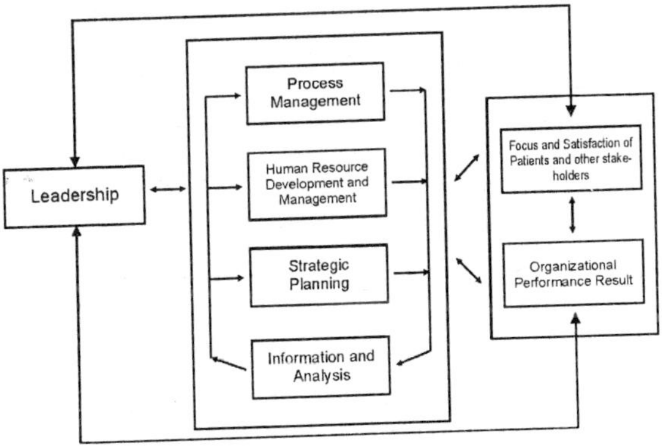

Further, MBNQA is based on the premise that management leadership and customer/external focus are two key factors in determining the efforts to introduce total quality. The EQA is rather explicit on the external focus in that the examination items dealing with customer satisfaction, and the requirement for the applicants to provide evidence of benchmarking. These awards clearly stress the role of customer and that the goal of quality improvement is customer satisfaction (Ghobadian and Woo, 1996). In the EQA model, the criteria are divided into two groups: enablers and results, the latter highlighting how the results are achieved in an organization. Counte and Meurer (2001) examined the Baldrige, King's Fund and EFQM award categories and identified seven categories which can be considered as additional, namely innovation, product control, contract requirements, inspection/audit and servicing. Many national quality awards are directly based on MBNQA and there is a lack of rigorous empirical testing on the causal relationships among criteria in healthcare in different countries.

Figure: 9.2

Relationships among EQA Criteria

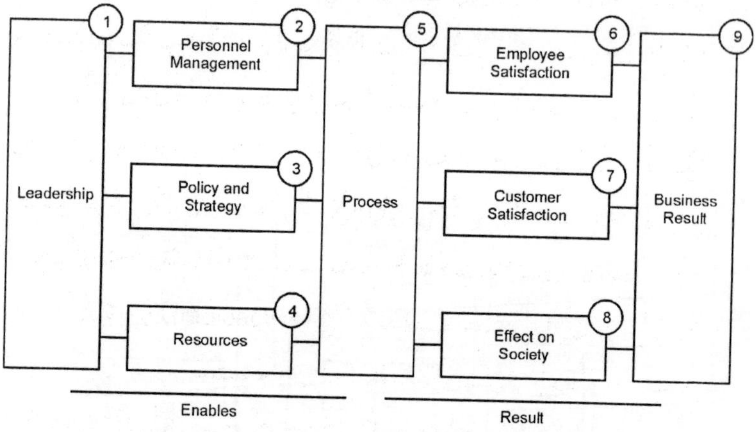

After a thorough review of the prescriptive, conceptual, practitioner and empirical literature on TQM and TQS spanning over 100 articles, Sureshchandar et al. (2001a) identified 12 dimensions of quality management as critical for the institution of a TQM environment in service organizations. The factors are: top management commitment and visionary leadership; human resource management; technical system; information and analysis system; benchmarking; continuous improvement; customer focus; employee satisfaction; union intervention; social responsibility; servicescapes; service culture. Based on literature evidence and logical reasoning, the various functions executed by these dimensions are portrayed by means of a conceptual model (Figure 9.3).

Figure 9.3

Conceptual Model of Total Quality Service

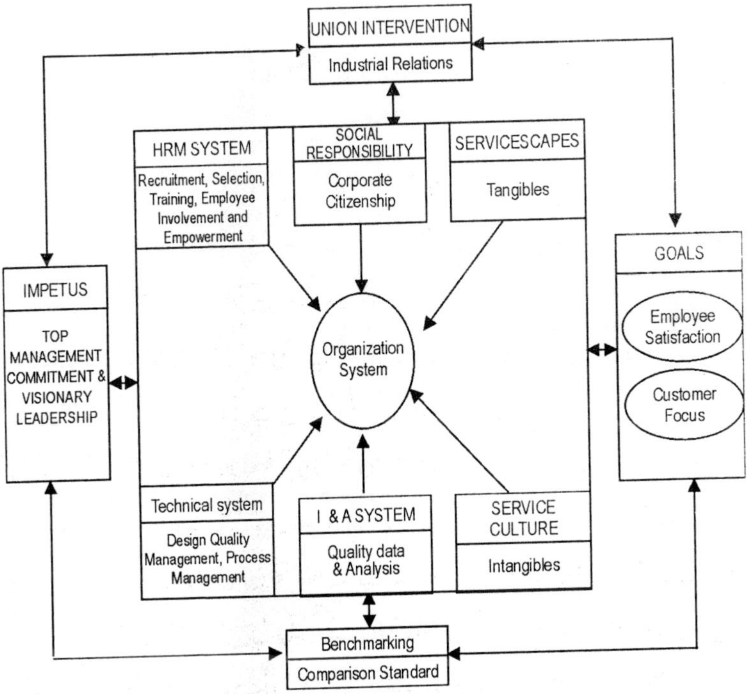

Source: Sureshchandar et al., 2001a, p. 356.

Kanji and SÁ (2003) presented an implementation plan of Kanji Business Excellence Measurement System (KBEMS). The model includes the following systems: leadership, delight the customer, management by fact, people-based management, continuous improvement, customer focus, process improvement, people performance, continuous improvement of culture and performance excellence. Figure 9.4 gives the diagrammatic representation of the model. Measurement techniques and performance evaluation are very crucial for evaluating organizational performance, and hence the authors have provided a detailed approach for measuring and arriving at an index. A final organizational performance excellence index (OPI) can be calculated which gives an aggregate measure of the excellence of the organization.

The authors have considered the KBEM as holistic and inclusive because of the following features:

- The whole system is driven by leadership and organizational values, which create a culture of improvement and coordination of efforts of all stakeholders.
- A realistic view of performance is made possible by involving internal and external stakeholders actively in the assessment process.
- Information sharing and cooperation among the various stakeholders are highlighted in the model.
- The main consideration is that of delighting the stakeholders, process excellence and organizational learning.

The authors have provided specific steps for the development of a measurement model for individual hospitals and data analysis for arriving at OPI. The model itself was not tested and validated by empirical research. The work lends support to the inclusion of performance measurement criterion for TQS framework for hospitals.

Chow-Chua and Goh (2002) identified a need to combine various models of performance measurement and quality improvement for healthcare sector and presented a knowledge-based framework for evaluating the performance of hospitals. The model integrated Singapore Quality Award criteria and the balanced score card (BSC) approach. The applicability of the

Figure 9.4

Kanji's Business Excellence Measurement System

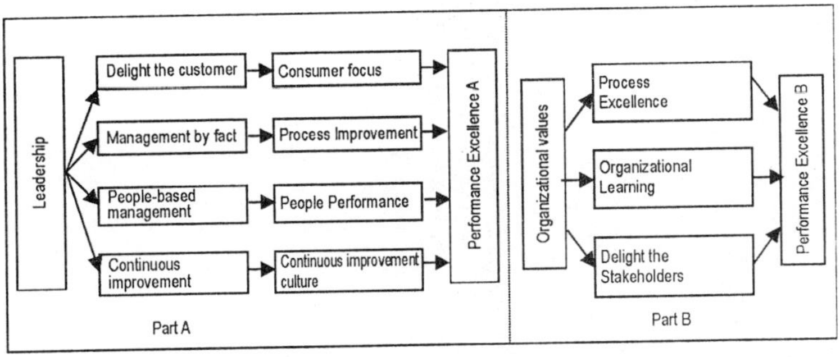

Source: Kanji and Sa, 2003.

Figure 9.5

Singapore Quality Award

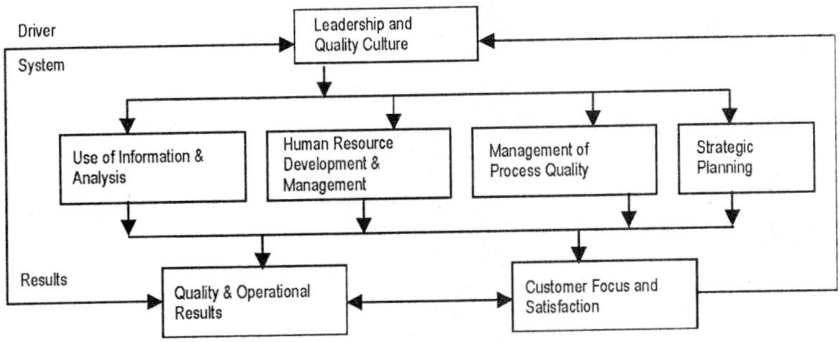

Source: Chow-Chua and Goh, 2002, p. 62.

model was illustrated using a case study of a public sector hospital in Singapore. The preliminary results showed a sustainable improvement in patient satisfaction and better inter-departmental communication. Based on the case study, the authors concluded that the integrated framework could help hospitals make better decisions based on structured measurement and knowledge. The Singapore Quality Award is based on MBNQA and Figure 9.5 shows the relationships among various quality criteria. This study further highlighted that integrating organizational performance and results criteria is important in a TQM model.

Lakhe and Mohanty (1994) studied various TQM conceptualizations of industries in order to provide an understanding of concepts, evolution and implementation of TQM. Taking into consideration the application of TQM in Japan, USA and Europe, they examined the quality issues in the developing nations. Inferring from the results of a case study of a manufacturing company in Bombay, they concluded that the organization considered TQM as most important for growth and success. Their case study highlighted the importance of service level offered to customers, poor quality products resulting in higher operating costs, training people in quality, incentives to be given to staff for quality work and top management commitment to quality. They argued that given the changes in the business world due to globalization, uniform quality standards are very important. Based on their case study findings and analysis, they suggested the following approach to TQM adaptation: Develop a vision, promote a policy on quality, create a total quality-oriented culture, and include training and education. They felt a national level all-out effort was required to bring about a major change in quality in industries and not just in individual organizations.

Using an intellectual and judgemental process of grouping similar requirements of quality management, Motwani (2001) identified seven critical factors and more than 45 performance measures of TQM based on extensive review of prescriptive, conceptual, practitioner and empirical literature. According to the author, the following seven-factor set, namely top management commitment, quality measurement and benchmarking, process management, product design, employee training and empowerment, vendor quality management and customer involvement and satisfaction captures the most important aspects of effective TQM. A possible sequence for implementation of factors with top management commitment as the base was recommended, followed by employee training and empowerment, quality measurement and benchmarking, process management, and customer involvement and satisfaction as pillars. Later, factors of vendor quality management and product design can be implemented to achieve TQM.

Insights gained from the above frameworks provided a base for developing a conceptual framework defining the relationships among the 13 quality constructs of this research. For studying the relationships among the constructs, the strength of correlation between the constructs were analysed.

TQS Constructs and their Relationships

The results of the research validated the criticality of the 13 constructs of the TQS model based on the implementation levels of reputed hospitals in the country with the help of a cross-sectional survey. In order to understand how these constructs are related to each other, it was decided to carry out a bivariate correlation (Pearson's Correlation) analysis. From the respondent set, the Senior Managers who were involved in quality activities/committees were interviewed about the various strategies they adopt for quality management and finally asked to rate the performance level among under each quality management strategy in comparison to the best practice in the industry. A five-point Likert Scale was used for the purpose. The rating scale used is as follows: 1-Worst in the industry; 2-Below Average; 3-Average; 4-Above Average and 5-Best in the industry. A total of 22 managers participated in this study and the ratings for each construct (13 in all) were noted.

The results are tabulated in Table 9.1. It is of interest to note from the ratings that the managers rarely rated the performance as excellent for all quality management strategies and hence were realistic in their assessment. The mean scores of the constructs indicate that the perceived performance level of all hospitals in the sample is high. The standard deviations do not show unusual data deviations and are judged to be reliable.

Table 9.1 clearly shows that all the correlations among the constructs are positive. This finding lends support to the notion that the TQS management strategies should be implemented holistically rather than piecemeal. Leadership and Management

Table 9.1

*Bivariate Correlation Matrices for 13 TQS Constructs**

	Mean	Std. D	L&MC	SP	HRM	HCS	PM	SC	SS	ADM	MIA	SQ	CF&S	KR	SR
L&MC	3.6818	.4767	1.000												
SP	3.6364	.4924	.701	1.000											
HRM	3.5455	.5097	.456	.459	1.000										
HCS	3.6364	.4924	.495	.411	.449	1.000									
PM	3.6364	.4924	.498	.411	.449	.607	1.000								
SC	3.6364	.4927	.295	.259	.269	.274	.411	1.000							
SS	3.5909	.5032	.424	.524	.269	.524	.716	.332	1.000						
ADM	3.4090	.5032	.370	.629	.273	.437	.437	.245	.504	1.000					
MIA	3.2727	.4558	.418	.251	.354	.351	.463	.251	.302	.321	1.000				
SQ	3.5909	.5032	.623	.332	.354	.524	.332	.140	.436	.428	.194	1.000			
CF&S	3.5909	.5032	.424	.332	.469	.446	.524	.524	.436	.504	.302	.260	1.000		
KR	3.5455	.5096	.748	.638	.267	.449	.449	.449	.354	.574	.559	.354	.540	1.000	
SR	3.4546	.5096	.428	.121	.467	.121	.500	.500	.203	.169	.466	.203	.388	.283	1.000

*All estimates of correlations are statistically significant at $p < 0.05$.

Legend: L&MC-Leadership and Management Commitment; SP-Strategic Planning; HRM-Human Resource Management and Development; HCS-Healthcare Services Design and Improvement; PM-Process Management; SC-Service Culture; SS-Servicescapes; ADM-Administrative System; MIA-Measurement, Information and Analysis; SQ-Service Quality Management; CF & S-Customer Focus and Satisfaction; KR-Key Results; SR-Social Responsibility

Commitment correlates well with all the constructs and therefore it can be seen as a necessary condition for ensuring various quality management strategies in a healthcare organization. The leadership in healthcare organizations is taking up a proactive approach and building systems and structures for quality. In the last two decades, the success of some of the corporate hospitals has been because of visionary leadership, professional management and allocating resources to establish appropriate mechanisms to deliver and improve technical as well as service aspects of care. It, however, shows a relatively low correlation with 'service culture' (0.295) which indicates that leadership and management commitment is a necessary condition but not a sufficient condition for achieving superior service quality. Changing habits and mindsets, and setting up a culture in order to achieve high quality of services take a long time. There is, however, a definite recognition and realization in that commitment from various groups of people in the hospital, which are essential for service excellence.

Strategic planning shows lower than desirable correlations especially with social responsibility. Presently, the hospitals are concentrating on developing their infrastructure and service capabilities. The main focus is establishment of business and making new projects viable. However, almost all hospitals from the study are found to be actually involved in some social cause such as health education, free camps (medical/surgical), adopting rural areas in the nearby vicinity, telemedicine to reach out to remote and lesser-serviced areas of the country, partnering with various national and international agencies for preventive care, etc. One specific example of partnerships is setting up of disaster management protocol by a consortium of multi-speciality hospitals in Bangalore for emergency situations. Many medical professionals agree that social responsibility inherent in medical services is more of a necessity for a country like ours.

Human Resource Management and Development is well correlated with Leadership and Management Commitment (0.456), Strategic Planning (0.459), Healthcare Service Design and Improvement (0.449), Customer Focus and Satisfaction (0.469), and Social Responsibility (0.467). This indicates that the HRM strategy of Human Resource Planning, Employee well-being and Empowerment and Training is very essential to TQS in hospitals. The strength of the hospitals in terms of high quality professionals are challenged by staff turn over (some hospitals reported nursing turn over rate as high as 40%) and training requirements. Managing people, their training and retention issues continue to be crucial in order to provide high quality services.

Healthcare Service Design and Improvement correlates very well with Process Management (0.607), Leadership and Management Commitment (0.498), Strategic Planning (0.411), Human Resources (0.449), Servicescapes (0.524), Administrative System (0.437), Supplier Quality (0.524), Customer Focus (0.446) and Key Results (0.449). These results also suggest a reinforcing impact of the critical role of Healthcare Service Design and Improvement (the technical quality) in attaining a superior overall service quality. Taking into consideration medical technology, patient requirements (age, disease stage, pattern, patient responses, etc.), procedural appropriateness, risk management, and constantly improving procedures and techniques based on accurate measurement are the crux of evidence-based medicine. Process Management (key and support processes) in fact shows one of the highest correlations with almost all other constructs (see Table 9.1) and this can be said to be in synergy with Healthcare Services which essentially determines how well services are delivered.

Customer Focus and Satisfaction, most important goal of any organization shows moderate levels of correlations with almost all constructs. Its relation to Supplier Quality is rather low (0.260, although more than statistical guideline of 0.25) and it is possible that the patients are not directly judging the quality of hospital supplies but would be interested in the overall services (technical and service aspects), whereas its relation to Healthcare Services would be crucial. The correlation values of Supplier Quality tend to support such a conclusion. Supplier Quality shows low correlation with Service Culture (0.140) and Measurement, Information and Analysis (0.194). It is not clear if it is because of lower implementation levels of the strategies by themselves or because the relationships themselves are of lower order.

> **Research Insights**
>
> Though all correlations are positive, importance of *Social Responsibility* in Total Quality Service Model needs to be further researched. There is a possibility of a stronger commercial orientation of healthcare organizations in general in the modern competitive world. As researchers and academicians, we strongly believe 'social equity and social-orientation' of hospitals is an essential aspect of 'total quality'. Under the pressures of economic viability and profit orientation, the managers may think otherwise. Indian government's interest towards 'Public Private Partnerships' in improving healthcare access to all would imply strong commitment from managers of private hospitals towards such an orientation.

Key Results of organizational performance are correlated well with almost all factors and it shows the importance of integrating key results into a TQS programme. Logically speaking, organizations will not implement quality as a strategy if it does not enhance the overall performance. Quality has become an important competitive strategy for long term survival. Interviews with a large number of experts and Senior Managers in the course of the research work confirmed such a notion. As one takes a closer look at Table 9.1, Social Responsibility is one factor that shows low correlations with Strategic Planning (0.121), Healthcare Services (0.121), Servicescapes (0.203), Administrative System (0.169) and Supplier Quality (0.203), respectively.

Measuring Instrument for TQS

As discussed in the earlier chapter, development of the *TQS measuring instrument* is based on a literature review and critical analysis of Quality Management research. Further, an in-depth analysis of QM practice as well as inputs from TQM experts were considered for improving the TQS instrument for hospitals in India. The constructs were empirically validated using survey data on QM strategies, actions and behaviours essential for achieving organization-wide excellence in quality. One hundred and forty-six Senior Managers of 29 major hospitals in India participated in the survey. The instrument developed in this research has high external validity for healthcare organizations, particularly for Indian hospitals as the sample included a wide range of hospitals in terms of size, level of service operations and a wide variety of services. Internal consistency is highest since it is applied to one industry and specifically designed for healthcare services.

Based on the research, 13 constructs for TQS framework were found reliable and valid, while four factors among them were further categorized into sub-factors based on Factor Analysis. The hypothesis is accepted with modifications implying that TQS framework is a 13-construct framework composed of the following constructs, with four of them having sub-factors:

1. Leadership and Management Commitment
2. Strategic Planning
3. Human Resource Management and Development *(Sub-factors: HR Planning; Training; Employee Well-being and Empowerment)*
4. Healthcare Service Design and Improvement *(Sub-factors: Healthcare Service Design; Healthcare Service Continuous Improvement)*
5. Process Management
6. Service Culture
7. Servicescapes
8. Administrative System *(Sub-factors: General Administration; Legal Administration)*
9. Measurement, Information and Analysis *(Sub-factors: Information and Analysis; Hospital Information System; Performance Management)*
10. Supplier Quality Management
11. Customer Focus and Satisfaction
12. Key Results
13. Social Responsibility

This TQS measuring instrument so developed can be used to measure the QM levels in hospitals. The instrument can be used for computing the TQS index (TQSI) for a hospital. The TQSI for a particular hospital with respect to a specific dimension is the average value (mean of the Executives scores say on a scale of 10) of all items in that construct, e.g., Likert Scale of 1 to 10 can be used to rate each question with 1 being 'not yet implemented' to 10 being 'fully implemented with highly successful results'. The TQSI will give an indication of the performance of a hospital with respect to a particular dimension. Decision-makers can use these indices as a baseline and implement continuous improvement by targeting higher levels of quality performance. Such indices would also help researchers to better comprehend the different facets of TQS in the healthcare sector in our country where quality management research is beginning to evolve. It can also be used as a basis for further studies in other healthcare organizations such as day clinics, primary health care clinics, etc. and in other countries.

TQS is a configuration and the QM strategies and their relationships are also important in that managers have to implement these in a holistic manner. Therefore, it was deemed important to test these relationships. Bivariate correlation analysis (Pearson's Correlation) was conducted for testing relationships among constructs with industry experts rating the performance level of their hospitals in comparison with the industry best practice. Positive correlations among the constructs indicted the interactive nature of the constructs. With this, an integrative framework for the TQS for hospitals is proposed.

Integrative Framework for TQS in Hospitals

An integrated approach to TQS in hospitals provides a framework within which managers/professionals can create a quality programme that enhances working life and services to patients. Such a programme is appropriate for the complex reality of the modern professional services and to the beliefs and abilities of the people who use and work in such organizations. From the results and discussion, it is clear that the proposed 13 constructs are critical for the establishment of TQS processes in hospitals. The 13-construct integrated structure for TQS aims to combine effective and established professional quality practices in a hospital with newer quality improvement methods while simultaneously improving customer and professional satisfaction.

These constructs have different functions in TQM movement in healthcare services. Based on literature evidence and logical reasoning, the various functions captured through these constructs are portrayed by means of a descriptive model as shown in Figure 9.6. The framework highlights the importance of technical, business and service orientation of healthcare providers. It provides a common language, simple methods and frameworks for professionals, managers and staff at all levels in the organization to work together to improve their services. It integrates the professional, management and patient-quality perspectives, and views the organization of services to a patient as a system made up of processes.

The following integrative framework for TQS for hospitals is proposed (Manjunath, 2010):

Leadership and management commitment act as a driver for TQS and continuous improvement. Their commitment should be translated into strategies for effective implementation of quality management in all areas of activities and in the whole organization. The top manager's role becomes one of motivating the professionals to want to improve quality, and ensuring that they know how to use organizational quality methods to understand and gain control over systems of care which they work in and contribute to. The focus of professional service management becomes managing patient/customer pathways, quality projects and co-coordinating development programmes, rather than 'managing personnel and operations' for one profession or department. Such a visionary leadership when combined with strategic planning based on objective data would drive the establishment of organizational system consisting of sub-systems of human resource management and development, service design, process management, administrative system support, physical infrastructure ambience (servicescapes), measurement, information and data analysis, and supplier quality management. Service culture system highlights the criticality of human behaviour especially in the interface of patients and families with

Figure 9.6

Integrative Framework for Total Quality Service in Hospital (Manjunath, 2010)

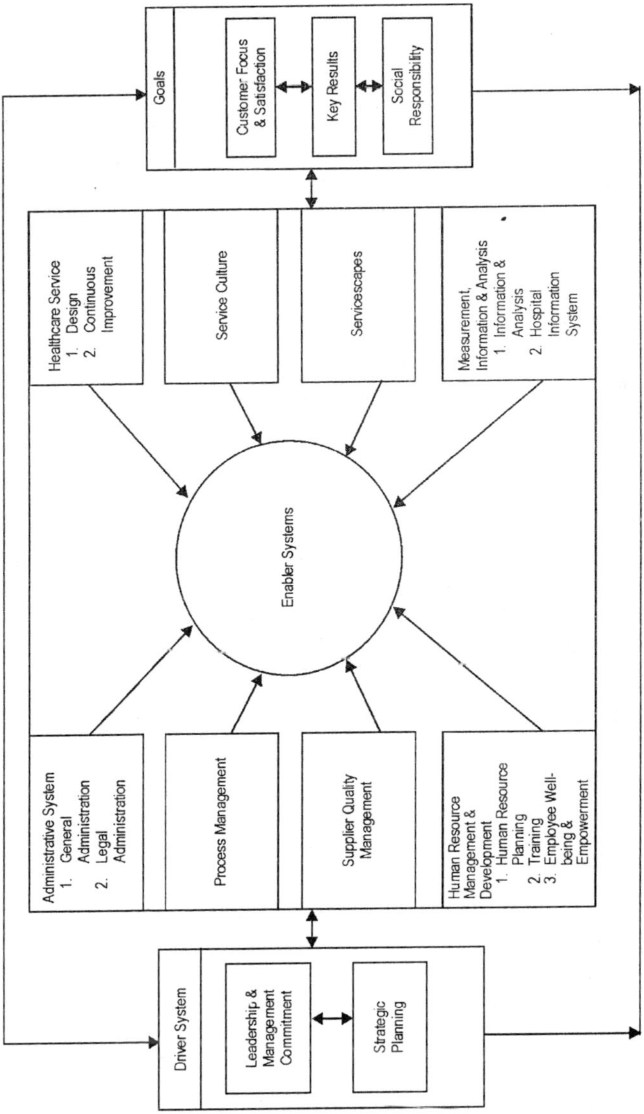

varied groups of healthcare providers within a healthcare service delivery system. Right set of attitudes of trust, openness, team spirit and a philosophy of 'right the first time' and 'right every time' among all employees sets the ambience of quality culture. In modern healthcare, quality depends not only on the competence of individual professionals but also on coordinated contributions of other employees. It depends on information and other systems that support the human interaction. Humility is needed in relating to patients, who are often well informed about what they require and expect a partnership with the professional, and in recognizing the need to learn and be able to use modern quality methods to understand and improve determinants of quality other than their own skill and knowledge. Such an integrated system can be viewed as an enabler of TQS in healthcare for achieving goals of customer focus and results with a social mission that healthcare services are naturally associated with. The customer focus and satisfaction form the basis of TQS and this along with key results are the goals that an organization would want to eventually achieve. The patient is the central focus of healthcare services as the psychology and actual participation of an individual patient (and families) determine not only how well the services can be provided but also the final outcome of care, namely, 'healing'. Impact on society and social responsibility of healthcare service provider is deemed as an important goal; the role of a leader in healthcare in ensuring healthier communities cannot be overlooked.

Summary

Various tested TQM models for services and healthcare are analysed and relationships among the criteria were synthesized. The relationships among 13-construct TQS framework were tested using bivariate correlation (Pearson's correlation) based on the ratings of quality performance on each construct in comparison to the industry best practice by 22 quality experts from the major hospitals. Positive correlations indicated that TQS constructs are interrelated and that the quality management efforts should be applied in a holistic manner rather than piecemeal.

Decision-makers can use this valid instrument for assessing quality performance and monitoring continuous quality improvement of hospitals. Researchers can use this instrument for studying Quality management of healthcare organizations. An integrative framework with 13 constructs for TQS management in hospitals is proposed in which Leadership and management commitment and strategic planning are the driver systems. Administrative System, Supplier Quality Management, Process Management, Human Resource Management and Development, Healthcare Service Design and Improvement, Servicescapes, Service Culture, Measurement, Information & Analysis are systems identified as enabler systems which managers implement as quality management strategies in all areas of hospital services. This would lead to high customer satisfaction, high performance in key result areas of the organization while fulfilling its social responsibility. These are the goals of management systems. The conceptual model of integrative framework for TQS in hospitals is schematically presented with driver, enabler and goals as three key systems. The TQS level of healthcare organizations and quality management effectiveness could be measured using the 118 items Measuring Instrument-TQS questionnaire (grouped appropriately under 13 quality constructs) and TQSIs for hospitals computed.

10

Conclusions and Future Research Directions

Growth in the healthcare industry since 1990s has been rapid and the health sector is one of the major key service sectors in 'India's Service Revolution'. Societies moving up on the scale of economic and social development are increasingly focusing on 'quality of life' enhancements through services such as public utility, government services, infrastructure, education, healthcare and so on. Basic requirement of any effective healthcare system is that it enhances average life expectancy and to improve quality of life and productivity. The focus of healthcare industry is also moving from 'curing and treatment of diseases' to 'wellness'.

Issues of funding, rising costs, utilization, consolidation, competition and quality along with political commitment dominated the healthcare sectors in the industrialized nations but in contrast a country like India struggles to increase its capacity to provide healthcare services to its huge population. The focus of management of a majority of hospitals in India can be thought, in broad terms, as shifting from 'expansion' to 'quality for survival' in a competitive environment and finally to 'quality excellence'. Achieving 'quality excellence' in the context of huge investments and rapid expansion of both public and private healthcare sectors in India in the backdrop of weak regulatory mechanism is highly challenging.

Quality in any sense is a comprehensive and multifaceted concept. Traditionally, healthcare services have been provider centric with professionals making major decisions about what is good for the patients owing to technical knowledge and expertise. Since quality has come to be recognized as a strategic tool for attaining operational efficiency and improved business performance of healthcare organizations, healthcare managers need to arrive at a more comprehensive definition of healthcare quality. Issues of technical aspects of quality as well as process and outcome quality, quality in fact and perception, and freedom from deficiencies and features are Critical. Finally, deducing from radical constructivism it was found that 'quality as a construct' would be a very useful approach for healthcare managers. This would help us define quality of healthcare services with various dimensions in order to address them adequately in quality management programmes.

Operationalization of the concepts of quality at the organizational level has led to several innovations in quality management, from the traditional Quality Assurance (QA) to implementation of the philosophy of Total Quality Management (TQM). Indian healthcare organizations, especially hospitals are using QA mechanisms such as ISO, NABH and JCI. Even though QA is a very important step in quality enhancements, long-term quality improvements and culture for quality is better ensured using the principles and practice of TQM. Quality Assurance provides conformance quality based on certain standards. In the context of liberalization, globalization, competition and consumer awareness, the healthcare organizations can no longer ignore quality of services they provide. Often, healthcare organizations are seen to move from inspection-oriented quality improvement system to one that orients itself to a systematic transformation of organizational culture through a comprehensive plan involving customer focus, key-process monitoring, data-driven tools, and techniques and team empowerment.

Contributions of the quality gurus, namely Deming, Juran, Crosby, Feigenbaum and Ishikawa have had a great impact on quality management of manufacturing and service industries. Similarly, the works of Donabedian, Berwick, Bluementhal, Kazandjian, McLaughlin, Kaluzny and others are of great interest to healthcare quality management. Evidence-based medicine, health technology assessment, customer orientation and cost-effective services are becoming important for every healthcare professional. Total Quality Management (TQM) known to manufacturing industry is an effective approach to quality improvement encompassing all systems and processes, clinical and non-clinical, with a focus on processes to improve the quality of all services and products for various groups of customers. A plethora of healthcare quality literature indicates that TQM in healthcare would work and result in enhancing the organization's overall performance as a healthcare provider as well as a business enterprise. For effective implementation of TQM in an organization, it is important to identify critical quality management strategies. The literature of QM implies that when decision-makers of an organization focus on better management of the critical factors, improvements in quality of products or services will occur. And ultimately, such efforts will result in improved organizational performance in terms of financial indicators, customer loyalty and satisfaction. Further, the researchers can use such operational measures to build theories and models for QM.

Research on critical success factors for TQM implementation in non-healthcare context is quite well established with a pioneering study by Saraph and others in 1989. Many researchers have identified the need for investigations of measurable variables associated with each of the TQM critical factors using data inputs from a large number of healthcare organizations to allow for generalisation. Majority of the factors extracted in the research studies correspond to quality award criteria, especially Malcolm Baldrige National Quality Award criteria. In fact, owing to the specific nature of needs of healthcare services, MBNQA has come up with healthcare quality criteria with suitable modifications (MBNQA, 2003). However, measurement of Organizational Performance and Results construct of MBNQA are not resolved and a need for more research on criteria other than the Baldrige categories and measures for implementation is identified. Empirical research by Kunst and Lemmink (2000) has also indicated that general application of European Quality Award (EQA) criteria as an evaluation instrument is debatable. Though the researchers can use the quality award criteria as a base for constructing TQM frameworks, conceptual theory building from extensive literature and expert inputs is essential in the healthcare services.

Sureshchandar and others in 2001 developed a holistic model for TQS and empirically validated the model using the survey method in the banking sector in India. Their model included service culture and servicescapes as important criteria for service sector and the importance of those factors in healthcare services is obvious. They recommended that the instrument could be used with necessary modifications for healthcare organizations. Healthcare specific elements such as epidemiological studies along with insurance payments and medical records data, involvement of the medical staff governance process (quality assurance methods such as peer review, hospital acquired infection committee, audit committee), risk-adjusted outcome measures (based on severity of illness, age, etc.), cost-effective analysis, use of quality assurance and risk-management data have to be incorporated in TQS of hospitals (McLaughlin and Kaluzny, 1999, pp. 8–10).

In the Indian context, professional management of hospitals is increasingly gaining importance since the 1990s, but research on TQS is very limited. Studies on implementation of QM strategies such as process management, patient satisfaction/expectation surveys, hospital infection rates and TQM in various hospital departments are reported. However, organization-wide implementation is a new phenomenon. At the hospital level, Tata Main Hospital, Jamshedpur, India, has implemented TQM. Tata Business Excellence Model (TBEM) based on the MBNQA criteria, formed the basis of the hospital's TQM implementation. Healthcare is highly fragmented and unorganized where nearly 85 per cent of hospitals are small (average bed strength 10). In general, quality of care among Indian hospitals varies quite considerably, and regulatory and accreditation mechanisms are quite new. So, it is difficult to accurately judge the quality levels of the hospitals. Therefore, the present study is an attempt toward further refinement of TQS constructs for the hospital sector from a managerial perspective.

Research Methodology and Analysis

The specific objectives of the study were:

- To identify quality dimensions critical to implementation of TQS in healthcare organizations.
- To develop an empirically tested, valid and reliable instrument for measurement of TQS for the hospital sector.
- To propose an integrative framework for TQS for hospitals.

The research on development of an integrative framework of TQS utilized the following methodology:

(i) Identification and selection of constructs for TQS in healthcare organizations was carried out from extensive literature review, analysis and synthesis.

(ii) Content validation of the TQS constructs was undertaken through expert inputs and analysis of quality management practices and performance of hospitals. This also provided a number of inputs and insights for developing and improving the measurement instrument for TQS. The studies are:

  (a) In-depth analysis of Senior Managers' inputs of a reputed hospital using case study research methodology was undertaken to measure the quality performance based on MBNQA healthcare criteria.

  (b) Expert survey was conducted to study the quality management practices in Indian hospitals using checklists and interview techniques.

(iii) Finally, an empirical research using cross-sectional survey of hospital managers in multi-facility (hospital) locations across India was conducted in order to validate the TQS measurement instrument. The managers rated the hospital's implementation levels on various factors of quality management using a Likert's scale. The data were analysed using SPSS package version 11.5. Confirmatory Factor Analysis (CFA) was applied, which seeks to determine if the number of factors and the loadings of measured (indicator) variables on them conform to what is expected on the basis of pre-established theory. Further, the correlations among TQS 13-constructs were tested based on the perceptual ratings of quality performance on each construct in comparison to the industry best practice by quality experts from the multi-speciality hospitals. Inferences were drawn based on the study results and an integrative framework of TQS management for hospitals was proposed.

From extensive literature review spanning over 100 articles in QM, organizational behaviour and healthcare quality research 13 TQS constructs were identified as critical to QM in healthcare organizations. The constructs so selected could be broadly classified under three categories:

1. The dimensions that are generic to QM of organizations belonging to different sectors but which have been extensively studied in the manufacturing sector and later found to be valid to services too including healthcare. These factors are Leadership and Management Commitment, Strategic Planning, Human Resource Management and Development, Process Management, Management of Information and Analysis, Supplier Quality Management, Customer Focus and Satisfaction, and Key Results.
2. The factors that need to be specially considered for service organizations, namely Servicescapes and Service Culture.
3. The factors which are critical to healthcare organizations, Healthcare Service Design, Administrative System and Social Responsibility are included as separate factors. The Patient Care Service Design (labelled as Healthcare Service Design in this research) is recognized specifically by MBNQA healthcare criteria. Administrative System is an important part of hospitals in terms of integrating various functions of a hospital and providing basic support to all operations. Social Responsibility was found to be a critical factor in the research by Kunst and Lemmink (2000) in healthcare and Sureshchandar et al. (2001a, b) in services. Also, healthcare is considered a social good and a basic right of individuals. Therefore the construct is included as a separate factor.

Content validity of the 13 TQS constructs for Indian hospitals was verified through expert inputs on quality practices and performance in hospitals. Using the case study research methodology, quality performance of a high achieving multi-speciality hospital located in a large town in South India criteria was carried out on the basis of MBNQA healthcare criteria. The results of this study indicated that though Baldrige criteria allowed quality performance evaluation in all areas, the managers of the hospital opined that Servicescapes, Service Culture and Administrative System can be included as separate factors. This case study research lent support to the appropriateness of the constructs selected from literature as critical to ensuring TQS in a hospital. Further, expert survey was conducted in order to understand the QM practices among hospitals through open-ended questionnaires and interviews of healthcare professionals/managers of some large hospitals in India. The content analysis of the information so gathered further strengthened the appropriateness of the 13 TQS factors identified through the review of literature. In addition, these two studies provided useful insights to revise and refine the TQS measuring instrument. The scales for the measurement model were determined and a questionnaire was developed for testing and validating the model. Thus, the TQS measuring instrument consisting of 118 items covering the entire range of organization-wide QM strategies for hospitals was developed after expert reviews and refinement.

In order to test the reliability and validity of the measuring instrument, a cross-sectional survey of hospital managers in multi-facility locations (hospitals) was undertaken. A total of 146 Senior Managers of 29 major hospitals from different regions in India participated in the survey. The managers rated each item on a five-point Likert Scale indicating the implementation level of QM strategy in their respective hospitals. Statistical analysis was carried out for the data collected using SPSS Version 11.5. The analysis included Cronbach's alpha coefficient for reliability, descriptive statistics for items (mean and standard deviation), Kaiser-Meyer-Olkin (KMO) Measure of Sampling Adequacy and construct validity for unidimensionality using CFA with the help of Principal Component Analysis. In general, item means for all constructs indicate an overall high average in the range of 3.55 to 3.98 and standard deviation around 1.0. All the constructs show KMO values more than 0.788 which indicated that the data set was suitable for Factor Analysis. Further, the constructs of the instrument were found to be highly reliable, with Cronbach's alpha α value in the range of is 0.7579 to 0.9392. Factor Analysis showed that the constructs explained 43.68 to 77.89 per cent variance, with Eigen values in the range of 1.56 to 5.18 and factor loadings on items in the range of 0.39 to 0.87. Nine constructs out of 13 were confirmed for unidimensionality and majority of the individual items showed factor loadings in the range of 0.6 and 0.8 which indicates the appropriateness of the items in the scales. Four constructs split into more than one sub-factors and were further subjected to reliability and validity analysis and were retained as valid constructs with sub-factors.

Using the Delphi expert consensus building technique, the sub-factors were labelled to ensure content validity. The split factors of four constructs were labelled as follows: Human Resource Management and Development (Sub-factors: HR Planning; Training; Employee Well-being and Empowerment); Healthcare Service Design and Improvement (Sub-factors: Healthcare Service Design; Healthcare Service Continuous Improvement); Administrative System (Sub-factors: General Administration; Legal Administration); Measurement, Information and Analysis (Sub-factors: Information and Analysis; Hospital Information System; Performance Management). Finally, the constructs were retained as originally constructed (with sub-factors) based on logical grouping of items and statistical analysis which indicated high Eigen values, factor loadings and per cent of variance in unrotated factor structure for all these factors.

The TQS instrument developed in this research is judged to have high external validity for healthcare organizations, particularly for Indian hospitals as the sample included a wide range of hospitals in terms of size, level of operations and variety of services. Internal consistency is highest since it is applied to one industry and specifically designed for healthcare services. The decision-makers and healthcare managers can use the instrument effectively to measure the quality performance levels of healthcare organizations. It is possible to rate the level of implementation for various dimensions and arrive at a TQS index (TQSI) for a hospital.

Further, the relationships among 13-construct TQS framework were tested using bivariate correlation (Pearson's Correlation) based on the ratings of quality performance on each construct in comparison to the industry best practice by 22 quality experts from the major hospitals. Positive correlations (ranging from 0.121 to 0.748 statistically significant at $p < 0.05$) indicated that the TQS constructs are interrelated and that the quality management efforts should be applied in a holistic manner rather than piecemeal. Since Leadership and Management Commitment correlates well with all the constructs, it is judged to be a necessary condition for ensuring various QM strategies in a healthcare organization. Social Responsibility is one factor that showed lower order correlations with many factors, namely Strategic Planning (0.121), Healthcare Services (0.121), Servicescapes (0.203), Administrative System (0.169) and Supplier Quality (0.203). The importance of Social Responsibility from a managerial perspective needs further investigation.

An integrated approach to TQS in hospitals provides a framework within which managers/professionals can create a quality programme that enhances working life and services to patients, a programme which is appropriate for the complex reality of the modern professional services and appropriate to the beliefs and abilities of the people who use and work in such organizations. These constructs have different functions in TQM movement in healthcare services. Based on literature evidence and logical reasoning, the various functions executed by these constructs were portrayed by means of an Integrative Framework as shown in Figure 9.6. A framework consisting of 13 constructs for TQS management in hospitals was proposed in which Leadership and Management Commitment and Strategic Planning form the driver system. Administrative System, Supplier Quality Management, Process Management, Human Resource Management and Development, Healthcare Service Design and Improvement, Servicescapes, Service Culture, Measurement, Information and Analysis are systems that enable managers to implement quality management strategies in all areas of hospital services achieving highest level of Customer Focus and Satisfaction. This would produce high performance in the organization's Key Result areas while fulfilling the Social Responsibility.

Specific Contributions of the Research

The present study is an attempt toward further refinement of Total Quality Service constructs for the hospital sector from a managerial perspective. The research has identified a comprehensive list of TQS management constructs addressing a wide (an entire) range of dimensions of QM in healthcare organizations. It is obvious that healthcare services will be dominated by professional services and technical quality is the core concern with procedural appropriateness, risk management and evidence-based practice of medicine. At the same time, TQS model for hospitals has rightly incorporated the business orientation essential for survival in an ever changing, competitive environment wherein cost effectiveness of services, value for money and profitability cannot be overlooked. Design and management of healthcare services with inputs from professional and patient (and family) interface, process management and information analysis along with a strong support form administrative and regulatory mechanisms in place (quality assurance/committees) would provide hospitals with a proactive approach in ensuring the highest technical quality. The constructs represent the human and non-human aspects of service production, delivery, facility tangibles and amenities to enhance the hygiene, comfort and the aesthetics aspects, supplier quality, data analysis and impact on the society. A culture of quality and service involving all and recognizing/rewarding various groups of employees appropriately is essential for integrating extremely complex healthcare services a modern hospital provides with a touch of care and concern. Training and human resource development occupies an important place in a highly human intensive service such as healthcare services. The framework therefore rightly takes care of management at internal organizational level, aligning its resources and activities to meet the industry, customer and society's expectations or demands. This would all be possible if and only if the leadership has long-term vision, planning and commitment to provide the highest quality services to its customers. Customer satisfaction, organizational performance in terms of key results and social responsibility are the combined goals of quality services of an organization.

The strength of the TQS framework is based on an extensive literature review and a synthesis of academic and practitioner QM literature in healthcare as well as non-healthcare environments. This research incorporated the general QM constructs from the empirical works by Saraph et al. (1989); Ahire et al. (1996); Black and Porter (1996); Ang et al. (2000); Zhang et al. (2000) and service specific ones based on the research by Sureshchandar et al. (2001a, b). Further, it included the healthcare specific elements based on the analysis of research by Huq (1996); Kunst and Lemmink (2000); and Meyer and Collier (2001). Comparing the study results with those of the recent studies in the Indian sub-continent context, the importance of the following factors for TQS are supported: service orientation (Andaleeb et al., 2007), patient satisfaction and loyalty (Raja et al., 2007; Naidu, 2009; Narang, 2010) and culture (Rabbani, 2009).

In the area of QM in healthcare, the empirical validation of the measurement instrument for TQS strives to enrich the subject of theory building using a multi-disciplinary approach. An Integrative Framework for TQS for Hospitals has been proposed which portrays the relationship among the constructs. The empirical research and statistical analysis lend credence to the so developed framework based on the criticality of the constructs chosen. The decision-makers and healthcare managers can use the instrument effectively to measure the quality performance levels of healthcare organizations. It is possible to rate the level of implementation for various dimensions and arrive at a TQS index (TQSI). Healthcare administrators and managers could use this framework for identifying areas of strengths and weaknesses in QM and continuously improve quality of services in a holistic manner.

This research work adds to the healthcare QM literature especially in the Indian context where there is a paucity of research. This would henceforth provide researchers and practitioners with objective information in the field of TQS that would enhance the understanding of intricacies and relevance of the various aspects of TQS in healthcare in different cultures and economies.

Limitations of the Study

The major limitations of the study are:

- CFA has shown that the 13-factor structure for TQS in hospitals is valid but four of the factors did not meet the criteria of unidimensionality but were composed of sub-factors. There is a possibility of confounding of factors in the four constructs, namely Human Resource Management and Development, Healthcare Services Design and Improvement, Administrative System and Measurement, Information and Analysis. However, it is important to note that the sub-factors under these formed homogenous groups of quality management strategies based on reliability and validity analysis. Labelling procedure for content validity based on expert consensus building through Delphi does support the decision to retain them under the construct originally selected. Further research is needed to re-examine the construct validity.
- Though the underlying theme of the TQS measurement instrument addresses the issues of hospitals in general, the study has been confined to Indian hospitals. There is a possibility of cultural bias as the expectations of people in a developing economy may be different than those of developed economies. Further research is indicated to evaluate this 13-construct TQS framework with larger and varied sample size in India as well as in other economies.

Future Scope of Research

- In order to improve external validity of the instrument, additional studies can be conducted with increased sample size, geographical diversity and various company/hospital types. Hospitals had started implementing NABH standards around the time the data collection for this research was nearing completion and therefore, NABH accredited hospitals could be sampled for testing and improving quality frameworks.

- The TQSI suggested in the study can be directly computed for even smaller hospitals (such as nursing homes and hospitals with less than 100 beds), which would throw light on the quality performance levels of various groups of hospitals. Such studies can provide specific directions for continuous improvement strategies.
- Study of relationships among TQS constructs in this research using bivariate correlation (Pearson's Correlation) indicated positive correlations among the 13 constructs. This supported the interactive nature of the QM strategies. Further, establishing the causal relationships through path model analysis for various criteria can be carried out using Structural Equation Modelling. Also, application of Analytical Hierarchy Process by assigning of weights to various quality constructs by healthcare quality experts could be explored. This would help in providing directions to managerial decision-making for prioritizing strategies and resources in order to achieve quality excellence.

In general, healthcare quality is a major emerging area in India, and systematic research and publication in this area would provide the much needed knowledge enhancements in order to implement QM strategies for performance excellence in the sector. Latest trends in QM through ISO Certification, NABH, Six Sigma and other Quality Models in hospitals and other healthcare organizations need to be explored and researched.

Appendices

APPENDIX A

Quality Management in Hospitals/Healthcare Organizations

Name (optional): Educational Qualification:

Designation:

Your phone number and e-mail id:

Name of the Hospital:

City/Town:

Website if any:

1. Describe your organizational profile in brief: (Please include information if your organization is Charitable, Service Oriented, Corporate, etc., the major services it provides, average number of Out-Patients seen per day, bed strength, etc.)
2. What are your major technologies, equipment, facilities? Mention special centres if any?
3. Describe major challenges for your organization in the next five years (from competitors, disease trends, resources, etc.).
4. Write your Organization's:
   - Vision
   - Mission
   - Core Values
5. Does your organization have a Quality Policy? If 'yes' please write it down.

6. Please mention which of the following Quality Management Programmes/Systems your organization uses. Describe briefly how such Programme are run.
   - *Programme/System Used (Tick the ones your organization uses).*
     - ❑ Quality Assurance Dept
     - ❑ ISO 9000
     - ❑ Accreditation
     - ❑ Kaizen (Suggestion Schemes)
     - ❑ Quality Circle
     - ❑ Benchmarking
     - ❑ Process Management
     - ❑ Medical Audit
     - ❑ Peer Review
     - ❑ Performance indicators (Hospital Infection Rates, Mortality, Morbidity Rates, Bed Occupancy, Cost, etc.)
     - ❑ Customer Satisfaction Surveys
     - ❑ Employee Satisfaction Surveys
     - ❑ 360 Appraisal System
     - ❑ Any other (please specify):
   - *Write details 'How does your organization apply the above programme/s?'*

   Describe the methods, tools and techniques used to follow the above programme/s: (Documentation, medical record checks, statistical quality control techniques, information/data analysis, brainstorming, training in quality, process improvement, cause–effect diagrams, standard operating procedure, etc.)
7. What according to you are the major problems/hurdles in achieving high quality of services in your organization?
8. Please feel free to provide additional inputs with specific reference to 'Quality' in Healthcare/Hospital in the space below.

   Thank You for Your Valuable Time and Inputs.

APPENDIX B

Survey Questionnaire

Quality Measures for Healthcare Organizations

I. Name of the Hospital:

Hospital (Mention Corporate, Private Ltd., etc.):

Service Type: Multi-specialty/Super-specialty/Specialty care/Others specify:

No. of Employees:

Turnover (in Crores of Rupees):

Growth Rate (in percentage):

Key Success Factor of the Hospital:

Does the Hospital have Performance Measurement System: Yes/No

Mention the system: Balanced Score Card/Performance Measurement Matrix/Other:

II. Instructions for filling the questionnaire

Please read each statement and *indicate the actual level of practice in your hospital* according to the scale anchor mentioned here. *Circle the number* corresponding to your rating for each statement.

Scale Anchor:

1. **Not at all**
2. **Occasionally**
3. **Somewhat**
4. **Frequently**
5. **Always**

A typical example is shown below:

1	2	3	(4)	5

Our focus on patients originates from within the management.

S. No.	*Items*	*Not at all*	↔			Always
1. Leadership and Management Commitment						
1.	Our senior executives are involved in quality activities.	1	2	3	4	5
2.	Our senior executives focus on improving patient care.	1	2	3	4	5
3.	Our senior executives are accessible to patients.	1	2	3	4	5
4.	Our senior executives set strategic directions for our hospital, such as deciding which new services to offer.	1	2	3	4	5
5.	Our department heads are responsible for leading quality improvement in their departments.	1	2	3	4	5
6.	The top management has inclination to allocate adequate resources and time for quality improvement efforts.	1	2	3	4	5
7.	Our employees can articulate the hospital's mission.	1	2	3	4	5
8.	Our focus on patients originates from within the management.	1	2	3	4	5
9.	We use performance feedback to improve the quality of care.	1	2	3	4	5
2. Strategic Planning (Long term planning and implementation)						
1.	Our strategies address both short-term and long-term planning.	1	2	3	4	5
2.	Our strategies address performance as both a healthcare provider and a business enterprise.	1	2	3	4	5
3.	Our strategies are translated into actions.	1	2	3	4	5
4.	Partnerships with other businesses support our strategic plans.	1	2	3	4	5
5.	Strategic decisions are evaluated with objective measures.	1	2	3	4	5
6.	Strategic plans are translated into specific requirements for each work unit or department.	1	2	3	4	5
7.	Our strategic plans include reducing waste (including rework, idle time, materials, etc.) in all departments.	1	2	3	4	5
8.	Long-term strategies include projections of how our services compare with key competitors.	1	2	3	4	5
3. Human Resource Management and Development						
1.	We align human resource plans with our organization's strategy (such as ensuring a proper mix of professionals).	1	2	3	4	5

Cont'd...

Cont'd...

2.	We derive employee hiring and development objectives from strategic objectives.	1	2	3	4	5
3.	Labour/Management relationships are cooperative.	1	2	3	4	5
4.	We motivate employees by improved job design (such as cross-training, job rotation, etc.).	1	2	3	4	5
5.	Employees are given a broad range of tasks.	1	2	3	4	5
6.	Frontline employees are trained on how to handle service failures ('recoveries' from patient property theft, long waiting times, etc.).	1	2	3	4	5
7.	Employees are rewarded for learning new skills and improved performance.	1	2	3	4	5
8.	We use training to build the capabilities of our staff.	1	2	3	4	5
9.	Employees are given decision-making responsibility.	1	2	3	4	5
10.	Employees including physicians are trained and encouraged for team involvement in quality improvement.	1	2	3	4	5
11.	We evaluate the benefits of staff training by measuring changes in skills or behaviour.	1	2	3	4	5
12.	Our work environment supports the well-being and development of all employees.	1	2	3	4	5
13.	We use a variety of methods to measure employee satisfaction (such as employee satisfaction survey, informal feedbacks, etc.).	1	2	3	4	5
14.	We work to improved employee health and safety (such as needle stick injuries, ergonomic training for jobs requiring lifting, handling of hazardous materials, etc.).	1	2	3	4	5
15.	Employees receive career development services.	1	2	3	4	5
16.	Employee turnover is evaluated in each department.	1	2	3	4	5
4. Healthcare Services Design and Improvement						
1.	New and revised healthcare services are reviewed and tested before they are introduced to patients (including new technologies).	1	2	3	4	5
2.	Patient preferences are analysed when designing new and revised patient services.	1	2	3	4	5
3.	Performance standards for new services are addressed during the design phase.	1	2	3	4	5
4.	Design requirements are considered by all appropriate departments to ensure integration (including advanced medical technology).	1	2	3	4	5

Cont'd...

Cont'd...

5.	Our service design process is continuously improved (using advanced technologies, medial research, etc.)	1	2	3	4	5
6.	We evaluate services on the basis of efficiency, including cost and timelines.	1	2	3	4	5
7.	We evaluate services on the basis of effectiveness, including appropriateness and risk.	1	2	3	4	5
8.	Procedures and possible outcomes are explained to patients so they know what to expect.	1	2	3	4	5
9.	Measurements/observations of patient services will indicate when corrective actions are needed.	1	2	3	4	5
10.	Our hospital uses a number of patient healthcare results/indicators for evaluation of services (patient length of stay, unplanned readmissions, disease-specific mortality rates, etc.).	1	2	3	4	5
11.	Clinical outcomes are measured and monitored internally (e.g., medical record checks, peer review, case discussion, medical audit, etc.).	1	2	3	4	5
12.	Clinical outcomes measurement and analysis is used to improve procedures, continuous learning, etc.	1	2	3	4	5
5. Process Management						
1.	We have standardized, simplified and documented service delivery processes (such as standard operating procedures, department protocols, etc.) for many key processes.	1	2	3	4	5
2.	We keep track and maintain the key processes that are critical to the business.	1	2	3	4	5
3.	Our hospital department protocols are well developed and documented.	1	2	3	4	5
4.	Systematic procedures for investigation of causes of errors and subsequent corrective actions are established.	1	2	3	4	5
5.	We emphasize on developing procedures for reducing the overall service-delivery times.	1	2	3	4	5
6.	We use a number of ways to improve our care delivery processes (use brainstorming, group discussions, etc.).	1	2	3	4	5
7.	All requirements (internal and external) are addressed in the design of support services (lab tests, housekeeping, medical records, pharmacy, etc.).	1	2	3	4	5
8.	We measure the performance of our support services and improve further.	1	2	3	4	5

Cont'd...

Cont'd...

9.	We obtain feedback on support services from patients and improve further.	1	2	3	4	5
6. Service Culture						
1.	All the employees realize that the real purpose of their work is 'service to patients/customers'.	1	2	3	4	5
2.	We have trust, openness and good relationships among the employees.	1	2	3	4	5
3.	Our employees have a strong belief in the philosophy of 'right the first time' and 'right every time'.	1	2	3	4	5
4.	Our employees have strong feelings such as 'My hospital', 'we work toward the hospital's excellent performance, image and customer service'.	1	2	3	4	5
5.	A strong 'team spirit' is highly prevalent among employees.	1	2	3	4	5
7. Servicescapes						
1.	The hospital ensures that there is a positive impact of the prevailing physical environment on patients/customers.	1	2	3	4	5
2.	The ambient conditions of the hospital are comfortable to customers (temperature, ventilation, noise, etc.).	1	2	3	4	5
3.	The signboards, symbols, advertisements boards, pamphlets and other artefacts in the hospital are appealing to the customers.	1	2	3	4	5
4.	The equipment, physical facilities and the materials associated with services are appealing to the customers.	1	2	3	4	5
5.	Housekeeping of the physical environment is kept as a priority of the highest order in the hospital.	1	2	3	4	5
6.	Physical environment, furnishings and equipment facilitate interactions with customers well.	1	2	3	4	5
8. Administrative System						
1.	We have integrated clinical and administrative services well.	1	2	3	4	5
2.	Both patient-and employee-related administration procedures are planned, documented and executed well.	1	2	3	4	5
3.	Feedback on administrative services is obtained form internal customers (other departments).	1	2	3	4	5
4.	Feedback on administrative services is obtained from external customers (patients and other stakeholders).	1	2	3	4	5

Cont'd...

Cont'd...

5.	Our hospital utilizes a number of financial and cost indicators to evaluate performance (inventory, investment, employee productivity, personnel/administrative costs, rate of increase in total costs).	1	2	3	4	5
6.	We monitor regulatory reviews of various committees (ethics, hospital acquired infection, quality council, etc.).	1	2	3	4	5
7.	We maintain licensure of hospital employees, registration, accreditation and comply with necessary regulatory mechanisms (for, e.g., NABL, ISO).	1	2	3	4	5
8.	The legal aspects of care and other management/administrative procedures are streamlined and backed by data/appropriate documentation (such as medico-legal cases, employee complaints, disputes).	1	2	3	4	5
9. Measurement, Information and Analysis						
1.	Our information systems are standardized across departments (patient care, accounting, etc.).	1	2	3	4	5
2.	Our information systems are integrated across departments.	1	2	3	4	5
3.	Both data collection and storing (hardware and software) are reliable and effective.	1	2	3	4	5
4.	Information systems are used to link caregivers' actions with patient outcomes.	1	2	3	4	5
5.	We have adequate sources of benchmarking information.	1	2	3	4	5
6.	We use benchmarking information to identify areas that need improvement.	1	2	3	4	5
7.	We have information on 'best-of-class' performance by our competitors for various hospital services.	1	2	3	4	5
8.	Organizational planning is based on objective data, which we have collected and analysed.	1	2	3	4	5
9.	We use objective data to identify our competitive advantage.	1	2	3	4	5
10.	Our data analysis shows improvement in cycle times (reduced length of stay, reduced waiting times, etc.)	1	2	3	4	5
11.	Training costs can be linked to positive changes in performance (quality of patient care, productivity, etc.)	1	2	3	4	5
12.	We compare performance measurements with our competitors (such as comparing costs per disease grouping/ICD or diagnostic-related groups).	1	2	3	4	5

Cont'd...

Cont'd...

13	We use data to identify trends that help us set priorities in how our resources are used.	1	2	3	4	5
14.	We use a number of statistical tools to analyse data in a number of areas.	1	2	3	4	5
10.	**Supplier Quality Management**					
1.	We establish long-term relationship with suppliers.	1	2	3	4	5
2.	Quality is our most important criterion for selecting suppliers than just price.	1	2	3	4	5
3.	Suppliers are involved in designing new and revised services (e.g., medical equipment service and maintenance).	1	2	3	4	5
4.	We establish supplier-rating system.	1	2	3	4	5
5.	We provide clear specifications to suppliers.	1	2	3	4	5
6.	We educate suppliers regarding our requirements, and provide technical assistance to suppliers.	1	2	3	4	5
11.	**Customer Focus and Satisfaction**					
1.	Customer focus and quality are driving forces behind day-to-day operations.	1	2	3	4	5
2.	Our employees exhibit pleasing and courteous behaviour toward different groups of customers.	1	2	3	4	5
3.	We measure customer feedback accurately and regularly.	1	2	3	4	5
4.	Overall satisfaction of patients and loyalty is high.	1	2	3	4	5
5.	Customer grievance redressal has a well-developed set of procedures and processes.	1	2	3	4	5
6.	We provide easy access to information for patients and other stakeholders.	1	2	3	4	5
7.	We resolve patient complaints in one step (rather than transferring to someone else).	1	2	3	4	5
8.	We take immediate and appropriate steps to eliminate 'causes' of complaints.	1	2	3	4	5
9.	We monitor community health trends.	1	2	3	4	5
12.	**Key Results**					
	Indicate Hospital Performance 1-very low; 2-low; 3-Average; 4-high; 5-very high					
1.	Profitability.	1	2	3	4	5
2.	Increase in number of customers/patients.	1	2	3	4	5
3.	Reputation of the hospital.	1	2	3	4	5

Cont'd...

Cont'd...

4.	Employee performance and satisfaction levels are satisfactory.	1	2	3	4	5
5.	Patient care results are satisfactory.	1	2	3	4	5
6.	Launching new services successfully.	1	2	3	4	5
13.	**Social Responsibility**					
1.	We integrate public responsibility into performance improvement efforts.	1	2	3	4	5
2.	Our employees follow a formal code of ethics.	1	2	3	4	5
3.	We lead efforts to improve community services, including education and environmental programmes.	1	2	3	4	5
4.	We are prepared for community emergencies.	1	2	3	4	5
5.	We provide good service at reasonable price, but not at the expense of quality, to people from all walks of life.	1	2	3	4	5
6.	We have partnerships with other organizations to improve community health programmes.	1	2	3	4	5
7.	We measure the performance of our community health services.	1	2	3	4	5
8.	We provide free services to those who cannot pay.	1	2	3	4	5
9.	We actively participate in health education for different groups of customers.	1	2	3	4	5
10.	We address environmental health/pollution issues with appropriate measures (for, e.g., disposing biomedical/hazardous materials appropriately, training staff and other customers involved in disposal, etc.).	1	2	3	4	5

APPENDIX C

Results and Analysis of Split Factors

Tables C.1

Factor Loadings of Unrotated and Rotated (Varimax Rotation) for the Construct Human Resource Management and Development

Unrotated Component Matrix (a) Construct 3: Human Resource Management and Development

	Component		
	1	2	3
VAR032	.789		
VAR026	.769		
VAR030	.764		
VAR033	.739		
VAR024	.721		
VAR027	.721		
VAR021	.704		
VAR028	.678		
VAR025	.674		–.501
VAR022	.655		
VAR018	.636	.552	
VAR031	.612		
VAR029	.597		
VAR023	.579		
VAR020	.578		
VAR019	.515	.591	

Note: Extraction Method: Principal Component Analysis.

Three components extracted.

Rotated Component Matrix (a) Construct 3: Human Resource Management and Development

	Component		
	1	2	3
VAR029	.789		
VAR022	.618		
VAR030	.614		
VAR033	.598	.415	
VAR031	.588		
VAR032	.573	.526	
VAR027	.569		.557
VAR021	.566	.409	
VAR026	.563	.466	
VAR020	.561	.408	
VAR025		.794	
VAR024		.694	
VAR023		.613	
VAR028		.554	
VAR019			.825
VAR018		.484	.688
KMO	0.905	0.754	0.506
Cronbach's Alpha (α)	0.8963	0.7698	0.7006
Eigen Value	5.183	2.379	1.558
% Variance Explained	51.834 %	59.471 %	77.891 %

Note: Extraction Method: Principal Component Analysis.
Rotation Method: Varimax with Kaiser Normalization.
Rotation converged in 10 iterations.

Table C.2

Factor Loadings of Unrotated and Rotated (Varimax Rotation) for the Construct Healthcare Service Design and Improvement.

Unrotated Component Matrix (a) Construct 4 Healthcare Service Design and Improvement

	Component	
	1	2
VAR039	.743	
VAR036	.742	
VAR042	.726	
VAR034	.723	
VAR038	.695	
VAR035	.683	
VAR040	.672	
VAR037	.665	
VAR041	.630	.514
VAR043	.589	.516
VAR044	.570	.426
VAR045	.569	

Note: Extraction Method: Principal Component Analysis.

Two components extracted.

Rotated Component Matrix (a) Construct 4 Healthcare Service Design and Improvement

	Component	
	1	2
VAR036	.820	
VAR035	.761	
VAR037	.748	
VAR038	.713	
VAR034	.699	
VAR039	.541	.512
VAR040	.505	.445
VAR041		.798
VAR043		.773
VAR044		.692
VAR042		.670
VAR045		.410
KMO	0.833	0.794
Cronbach's Alpha (α)	0.8659	0.7707
Eigen Value	3.892	2.685
% Variance Explained	55.605	53.698

Note: Extraction Method: Principal Component Analysis.

Rotation Method: Varimax with Kaiser Normalization.

Rotation converged in three iterations.

Table C.3

Factor Loadings of Unrotated and Rotated (Varimax Rotation) for the Construct Administrative System

Component Matrix (a)

Construct 8
Administrative System

	Component	
	1	2
VAR070	.797	
VAR068	.765	–.422
VAR069	.765	
VAR067	.760	
VAR066	.668	–.465
VAR071	.638	
VAR072	.633	.469
VAR073	.468	.741

Note: Extraction Method: Principal Component Analysis.

Two components extracted.

Rotated Component Matrix (a)

Construct 8
Administrative System

	Component	
	1	2
VAR068	.868	
VAR066	.813	
VAR067	.729	
VAR069	.701	
VAR070	.597	.535
VAR073		.875
VAR072		.750
VAR071		.592
KMO	0.839	0.642
Cronbach's Alpha (α)	0.8483	0.6790
Eigen Value	3.117	1.831
% Variance Explained	62.341%	61.025%

Note: Extraction Method: Principal Component Analysis.

Rotation Method: Varimax with Kaiser Normalization.

Rotation converged in three iterations.

Table C.4

Factor Loadings of Unrotated and Rotated (Varimax Rotation) for the Construct Measurement, Information and Analysis.

Component Matrix(a)

Construct 9
Measurement, Information and Analysis

	Component		
	1	2	3
VAR082	.843		
VAR079	.821		
VAR081	.777		
VAR087	.771		
VAR078	.761		
VAR086	.755		
VAR075	.745		
VAR080	.722		
VAR084	.721		.521
VAR074	.721		
VAR077	.719		
VAR076	.716		–.426
VAR085	.704		
VAR083	.702		

Note: Extraction Method: Principal Component Analysis.

Three components extracted.

Rotated Component Matrix(a)

Construct 9
Measurement, Information and Analysis

	Component		
	1	2	3
VAR086	.835		
VAR087	.727		
VAR081	.715		
VAR082	.636		.526
VAR076	.604	.595	
VAR080	.567	.413	
VAR074		.747	
VAR075		.744	
VAR077		.710	
VAR078		.684	.439
VAR079		.652	.601
VAR084			.825
VAR085			.745
VAR083	.477		.580
KMO	0.893	0.820	0.707
Cronbach's Alpha (α)	0.8992	0.8848	0.8082
Eigen Value	4.009	3.428	2.177
% Variance Explained	66.813 %	68.557 %	72.628 %

Note: Extraction Method: Principal Component Analysis.

Rotation Method: Varimax with Kaiser Normalization.

Rotation converged in six iterations.

Labelling of Sub-Factors

Delphi technique of expert opinion consensus-building process was used for choosing the most appropriate label for the sub-factors. The opinions of the experts in the field were sought. The experts consisted on three academicians (TQM experts) and five hospital managers in charge of quality management (ISO process/Medical Records-Medical Audit/TQM).

The steps followed were:

- *Problem was identified*: The problem was the selection of appropriate labels for items grouped by Factor Analysis (i.e., four factors which did not fulfil the unidimensionality criteria and split into more than one factor).
- *Expert opinion was sought:* It was anonymously and individually sought through a covering letter explaining the purpose and sending the items grouped in the same order by Factor Analysis. Each expert was requested to provide a label to each group of factors (i.e., 10 sub-factors under four factors in all) and return the data sheets.
- *Expert opinions were analysed:* All the labels for each sub-factor were sent back and each expert was asked to select the best title from those collected from the first round.
- Three rounds of the above process were carried out till a consensus was reached on the 'label of a factor'.

Based on the above processes, the sub-factor labels were arrived. The sub-factors under the main construct and the measurement items are given in Tables C.5, C.6, C.7 and C.8.

Table C.5

Scale Items – Human Resource Management and Development (Construct 3)

Factors	*Measurement Items*
Factor 1 Label Employee Well-being and Empowerment	1. Labour/Management relationships are cooperative.
	2. Employees are given a broad range of tasks.
	3. We motivate employees by improved job design (such as cross-training, job rotation, etc.)
	4. Employees are given decision-making responsibility.
	5. Employees including physicians are trained and encouraged for team involvement in quality improvement.
	6. Our work environment supports the well-being and development of all employees.
	7. We use a variety of methods to measure employee satisfaction (such as employee satisfaction survey, informal feedbacks, etc.).
	8. We work to improved employee health and safety (such as needle stick injuries, ergonomic training for jobs requiring lifting, handling of hazardous materials, etc.).
	9. Employees receive career development services.
	10. Employee turnover is evaluated in each department.
Factor 2 Label Training	1. Frontline employees are trained on how to handle service failures ('recoveries' from patient property theft, long waiting times, etc.).
	2. Employees are rewarded for learning new skills and improved performance.
	3. We use training to build the capabilities of our staff.
	4. We evaluate the benefits of staff training by measuring changes in skills or behaviour.
Factor 3 Label Human Resource Planning	1. We align human resource plans with our organization's strategy (such as ensuring a proper mix of professionals).
	2. We derive employee hiring and development objectives from strategic objectives

Table C.6

Scale Items –Healthcare Service Design and Improvement (Construct 4)

Factor 1 Label Healthcare Service Design	1. New and revised healthcare services are reviewed and tested before they are introduced to patients (including new technologies).
	2. Patient preferences are analysed when designing new and revised patient services.
	3. Performance standards for new services are addressed during the design phase.
	4. Design requirements are considered by all appropriate departments to ensure integration (including advanced medical technology).
	5. Our service design process is continuously improved (using advanced technologies, medical research, etc.).
	6. We evaluate services on the basis of efficiency, including cost and timelines.
	7. We evaluate services on the basis of effectiveness, including appropriateness and risk.
Factor 2 Label Healthcare Service Continuous Improvement	1. Procedures and possible outcomes are explained to patients so they know what to expect.
	2. Measurements/observations of patient services will indicate when corrective actions are needed.
	3. Our hospital uses a number of patient healthcare results/indicators for evaluation of services (patient length of stay, unplanned readmissions, disease-specific mortality rates, etc.).
	4. Clinical outcomes are measured and monitored internally (e.g., medical record checks, peer review, case discussion, medical audit, etc.).
	5. Clinical outcomes measurement and analysis is used to improve procedures, continuous learning, etc.

Table C.7

Scale Items – Administrative System (Construct 8)

Factor 1 Label General Administration	1. We have integrated clinical and administrative services well.
	2. Both patient-and employee-related administration procedures are planned, documented and executed well.
	3. Feedback on administrative services is obtained from internal customers (other departments).
	4. Feedback on administrative services is obtained from external customers (patients and other stakeholders).
	5. Our hospital utilizes a number of financial and cost indicators to evaluate performance (inventory, investment, employee productivity, personnel/ administrative costs, rate of increase in total costs).
Factor 2 Label Legal Administration	1. We monitor regulatory reviews of various committees (ethics, hospital acquired infection, quality council, etc.).
	2. We maintain licensure of hospital employees, registration, accreditation, and comply with available regulatory mechanisms (e.g., NBE, NABL, ISO).
	3. The legal aspects of care and other management/administrative procedures are streamlined and backed by data/appropriate documentation (such as medico-legal cases, employee complaints/disputes).

Table C.8

Scale Items – Measurement, Information and Analysis (Construct 9)

Factor	Items
Factor 1 Label Information and Analysis	1. Both data collection and storing (hardware and software) are reliable and effective.
	2. We have information on 'best-of-class' performance by our competitors for various hospital services.
	3. Organizational planning is based on objective data, which we have collected and analysed.
	4. We use objective data to identify our competitive strengths.
	5. We use data to identify trends that help us set priorities in how our resources are used.
	6. We use a number of statistical tools to analyse data in a number of areas.
Factor 2 Label Hospital Information System	1. Our information systems are standardized across departments (patient care, accounting, etc.).
	2. Our information systems are integrated across departments.
	3. Information systems are used to link caregivers' actions with patient outcomes.
	4. We have adequate sources of benchmarking information.
	5. We use benchmarking information to identify areas that need improvement.
Factor 3 Label Performance Management	1. Our data analysis shows improvement in cycle times (reduced length of stay, reduced waiting times, etc.).
	2. Input costs (investments) can be linked to positive changes in performance (quality of patient care, better patient care results, etc.).
	3. We compare performance measurements with our competitors (such as comparing costs per disease grouping/ICD or treatment procedures).

APPENDIX D

Explanation of Constructs

The detailed explanation of 13 constructs of TQS for healthcare is presented below. The importance of each construct in determining the overall quality is carefully examined from various studies and logical relationship among different management actions best representing each construct is analysed. Such an exercise helped establish the measurement items to be included for each construct.

1. Leadership and Management Commitment

The factor of 'Leadership and Management Commitment' is identified in almost all models of TQM including the quality awards of most countries. The crucial role of top management leadership in creating the goals, values and systems that guide the pursuit of quality improvement on a continuous basis cannot be missed by anyone. The understanding of Senior Managers that quality should receive a higher priority over cost or schedule and that in the long run, superior quality will lead to improvements in cost and delivery performance acquires special significance. A predominant theme in TQM literature is the role of top management commitment in terms of allocating resources, setting up systems, influencing and communicating the commitment to quality to all in the organization. Lin and Clousing (1995) surveyed the TQM practices in healthcare and found that top management lead the TQM efforts by putting a number of supportive systems in place such as training/education, administration, restructuring, communications and encouraging participation. The literature has consistently identified that lack of senior management commitment, fuzzy or unclear purpose or mission of organization and lack of appropriate resources of time, trained manpower and budget for quality activities would result in lack of consistency, alignment and integration of product or service quality (Gaucher and Coffey, 1993, p. 21; Short and Rahim, 1995; Aggarwal and Zairi, 1997; Nwabueze and Kanji, 1997; Zabada et al., 1998; Ennis and Harrington, 1999a, b; McLaughlin and Simpson, 1999, p. 34; Theodorakioglou and Tsiotras, 2000; Adinolfi, 2003; Kanji and SÁ, 2003). In an empirical study by Castle (1999) on various characteristics of top management, commitment and professional involvement were found to have a significant effect on the likelihood of adopting Quality Improvement in nursing homes (in the US).

Many models including MBNQA and EQA, in fact identify leadership and management commitment as a driver to quality improvement programmes in an organization. Based on the empirical evaluation of the causal relationships in the Baldrige Health Care Pilot Criteria, Leadership is identified as a driver of all components in the Baldrige System. Meyer and Collier (2001) concluded that the Baldrige theory 'Leadership drives the System which creates the Results' stands supported. Further, Kanji Business Excellence Model for healthcare depicts that the whole system is driven by leadership and organizational values which help create a culture of improvement and coordination of efforts of all stakeholders (Nwabueze and Kanji, 1997; Kanji and SÁ, 2003).

Based on the above analysis, the construct of Leadership and Management Commitment in this study is defined as a manifestation of: accessibility of senior leaders to patients, focus on improving patient care services and decisions to provide new improved services with an inherent focus on quality, resource allocation, involve everyone and constantly seek feedback to improve services. Commitment to quality then is not only a matter of conviction but also of a missionary zeal from top-level leaders down the management hierarchy. Leadership has to ensure employee participation, motivation and commitment to bring about the workplace transformation that TQM requires. Leaders as role models are important in healthcare set up. It means that the leaders have the capacity to learn from and adapt to change in an environment of openness and mutual trust that allows people to embrace change and experiment without feeling threatened (Applebaum and Wohl, 2000).

2. *Strategic Planning*

Along with leadership, strategic planning forms the key driver for quality performance. In the context of an ever-growing competition in the hospital sector, quality as a competitive strategy has become very crucial for hospitals and the top management has to address hospital performance as both a healthcare provider and a business enterprise. Long-term planning in terms of enhancing cost and resource efficiencies or waste reduction have become essential as the industry faces failures of healthcare organizations (Goonan, 1995; Huq, 1996; Ginter et al., 2002). Since hospital essentially depends on several other key players such as suppliers, diagnostic facilities and referral hospitals, collaborative programmes with national or international organizations in medical research, training and education, setting up quality programmes in place, etc., partnerships with other business enterprises is the key to continuously enhance the organizational performance. In fact, studies have shown that short-term orientation of administrators and managers, limited and poor translation of the strategies and goals into actions across various departments and lack of consistency, alignment and integration are barriers to successful TQM implementation (Gaucher and Coffey, 1993, p. 21; Short and Rahim, 1995; Aggarwal and Zairi, 1997; Nwabueze and Kanji, 1997; Zabada et al., 1998; Ennis and Harrington, 1999a, b; McLaughlin and Simpson, 1999, p. 34; Theodorakioglou and Tsiotras, 2000; Adinolfi, 2003; Kanji and Sa, 2003).

Many TQM frameworks essentially include the issues of strategic planning and implementation as a critical factor (Tables 4.1 and 4.2). Among the empirically tested models from literature, the following studies are worth mentioning to highlight the importance of strategic planning for achieving high levels of quality, they are: Black and Porter's (1996) Strategic Quality Management, Huq's (1996) Quality Mission Statement, Vision and Plan Statement of Zhang et al. (2000), Policy and Strategy of EQA (Kunst and Lemmink, 2000), Strategic Planning in MBNQA (Flynn and Saladin, 2001; Meyer and Collier, 2001) and Strategic Planning in Singapore Quality Award (Chow-Chua and Goh, 2002).

The construct 'Strategic Planning' measure in this study includes the organization's ability to develop and integrate short-

and long-term quality plans; address performance as a healthcare provider and a business enterprise; partnerships with others for support; implementation of plans to various work units; use of objective measures and plan for reducing ineffective ways and compare with key competitors to ensure long-term survival.

3. *Human Resource Management and Development*

People issues are occupying the most crucial position in management of organizations and rightly so. Role of human resources and importance of individual employee was hardly recognized by the classic quality 'gurus', namely Deming, Juran, Feigenbaum, Crosby and Ishikawa (Krüger, 2001). Though quality gurus such as Deming included training as an important factor in holistic quality management, motivating employees so that they dedicate themselves to work and other aspects of human issues has further evolved in TQM. The human factor has emerged as a critical one in both manufacturing and service industries particularly so in a highly sensitive and human intensive service such as healthcare.

Use of advanced technology in running an organization efficiently will not take away the importance of people. Human Resource (HR) and training factor measures the organization's ability to develop and realize the full potential of its workforce, including management, and to maintain an environment conducive to full participation, quality leadership and personal and organizational growth. In a service organization, the interaction between the service provider and the customer (patient and/or family) is so great that it determines the quality perceptions and satisfaction of the consumer. Employees play a crucial role in the production and marketing of healthcare services due to the nature of work in hospitals. Quality in healthcare is largely dependent on the understanding, behaviour and actions of the healthcare staff (doctors, nurses and others). Human actions in general are based on sensemaking in their present moment of experience. Making sense and meaning of life can be both in an individual and a collective perspective (Lindberg, 2002). This is so much true for TQM practices which require strong conviction and understanding to be effective in a hospital-wide context. Therefore, HR planning, bringing about change, continuous training and learning, involvement of staff at various levels are the essentials of success.

The HR planning is of strategic importance and proper mix of professionals and recruitment practices have to be streamlined with organizational strategic goals. Proper recruitment and selection of staff determines the quality of the workforce and their participation. This will eventually determine the quality of services any organization provides. Yang (2003) has highlighted the HR issues of shortage of physicians and problems of recruitment. Education and training is recognized as a very important factor for TQM practices in literature repeatedly. While studying the causal relationships among the Baldrige Health Care Pilot Criteria, Meyer and Collier (2001) found that Human Resource Development and Management and Process Management were significantly linked with Customer Satisfaction. Based on the comparison of empirically validated critical factors by various researchers, employee relations, training, development, empowerment, familiarity with TQM, participation and reward/recognition, and union intervention emerge as important components of Human Resource Management and Development in an organization. Lin and Clousing's (1995) study showed that support mechanisms for TQM success in hospitals included training/education support, reorganizations, encouraging participation, communications, and recognition and reward.

Empowerment of employees through knowledge, teamwork participation and decision-making participation would go a long distance in determining the high quality of services. Many good hospitals in fact provide a number of opportunities of learning for their staff particularly the medical staff in order to leverage the latest knowledge in the fast and ever-growing gamut of healthcare technologies. Brooks and Zeitz (1999) studied the perceived justice as a mediator between TQM dimensions and organizational commitment. It was found that provision of quality training enhanced procedural justice (openness and proper decision-making by supervisors). It is possible that professional employees value the opportunity for further training, which enhances their development as professionals. Lack of staff involvement particularly physician involvement has been identified as a major obstacle to TQM in hospitals by many researchers. Resistance by employees including physicians, nurses and other medical staff to change, physician autonomy and occupational sub-cultures have made implementation of TQM so much more difficult in healthcare (Gaucher and Coffey, 1993, p. 21; Short and Rahim, 1995; Aggarwal and Zairi, 1997; Nwabueze and Kanji, 1997; Zabada et al., 1998; Ennis and Harrington, 1999a, b; McLaughlin and Simpson, 1999, p. 34; Theodorakioglou and Tsiotras, 2000; Adinolfi, 2003; Kanji and SÁ, 2003). Another important area of human relations and involvement includes the union – management relationships (Short and Rahim, 1995). Sureshchandar et al. (2001a, b) included the Union Intervention as a separate factor critical to total quality in services. However, the factor showed a low correlation with other factors and it can be argued that it deserves to be considered as a part of human relations/involvement and development and not as a separate factor.

With a highly knowledgeable work force, hospitals face the challenge of motivating, retaining and rewarding employees. Training in soft skills such as communication skills, interpersonal relations, teamwork and customer service is emerging as important in the service sector (Sureshchandar, 2001a). Education and training so that staff sees a reason for change, understand the TQM philosophy, quality improvement processes, use of analytical tools, techniques and skills, and people skills are all highlighted in literature (Gaucher and Coffey, 1993, pp. 246–80). Ho (1999) reported that there is a need to train the staff so that they understand patient's psychology. Teams and problem-solving training were found to be associated with performance (Harrington, 1997).

Another important area is that of employee development and motivation for consistently high levels of performance and continuous learning. In general, Meyer and Collier (2001) have reported that developing better work systems, improving staff training, and measuring and promoting staff well-being, (all advocated by Baldrige criteria) should result in increased satisfaction of hospital staff, which in turn should improve patient (and other customers) satisfaction. From the above discussion, the construct of Human Resources Management encompasses HR planning, education/training and staff development including rewards, recognition and participation of all employees and emerges as highly crucial in providing TQS in hospitals.

4. Healthcare Service Design and Improvement

Designing services or products so that excellence in quality is achieved is emphasized in the TQM literature abundantly. Sound product design meets or exceeds the requirements and expectations better than the competitors. Before production, new product design should be thoroughly reviewed in order to avoid problems happening during production. In manufacturing literature, experimental design and quality function deployment are effective methods in product design (Zhang et al., 2000). Kaulio (1998) highlighted selected methods for Quality Function Deployment (QFD) involving the customers in three phases: specification, concept development and prototyping. Ahire et al. (1996) have emphasized the nature of complex products which require an interdisciplinary approach such as inputs from design engineer, manufacturing design team and marketing experiences to enhance the product quality at the design stage. Such methodologies are rather very well understood and implemented in product design and services continue to implement their service design through similar approaches. Works of Motwani (2001) and Silvestro (2001) highlighted the importance of service design in non-healthcare set up. Sureshchandar et al. (2001a, b) included service design as a part of technical system factor in which sound and reliable service design echoes an organization's strategic quality planning abilities and enables the organization to surmount customers' needs, expectations and desires, consequently, resulting in improved business performance. Two basic quality strategies can be identified, which when adopted would ensure high quality services from the design stage itself. One is prevention, that is, ensuring that the design of the service avoids quality problems arising during production and two, *zero fault strategy* which means when the design is right and employees do the right things, then the service would have zero faults. To achieve this in healthcare services, a number of medical and technological considerations are important.

Success of biomedical research and rapid diffusion of expensive high-tech medical procedures into daily practice have changed the way patient care services are designed. Such rapid pace of advancements necessitates that the hospitals and physicians/specialists introduce new methods of clinical care. West (2001) has acknowledged that it is quite appropriate that the most important focus of medical and nursing care is on individual patient care. Therefore, designing appropriate service would involve the technical aspects of care which refers to the accuracy of medical diagnosis and procedures, and conformance to professional specifications (Kanji and SÁ, 2003). Here, the appropriateness of medical technologies and then integrating it with patient needs becomes important. Technical aspects of patient/clinical care should involve risk management in terms of managing adverse events and medical errors (Boyce, 1997; Buchan, 1998; Sutcliffe, 2004). Chassin and Galvin (1998) have emphasized that the quality of healthcare should focus of technical quality of care and address the problems of overuse, underuse or misuse of procedures or medical technologies. Reducing overuse and misuse improves quality and reduces cost too. Appropriateness of procedures and medical errors should be measured and improved upon a continuous basis so that the clinical service is of high quality and cost effective.

Further, to ensure or minimize errors, a number of yardsticks (indicators) have to be identified, which when correctly measured aids continuous improvements in the services. A number of healthcare professionals have emphasized the importance of patient choice, patient preferences, expectations and involvement in designing and improving patient care services (Nwabueze and Kanji, 1997; O'Keeffe and O'Sullivan, 1997; Thomson and Hudgson, 1997; Ennis and Harrington, 1999; Köeck, 1999).

The MBNQA modified the general criteria framework to suit the specific needs of healthcare quality. Meyer and Collier (2001) validated the criteria of patient care service design, delivery and measurement for MBNQA healthcare criteria. From the above discussion the following features of *healthcare service design and improvements* emerge: the criticality of designing patient care services with procedural appropriateness taking into consideration the latest and advanced technology aspects (professional inputs) as well as patient needs and preferences as well as cost factors. Further, the services have to continuously improve based on evaluation of clinical outcomes, indicators of effectiveness, appropriateness and risk management.

5. Process Management

Management of core and support business processes is vital for effective quality enhancement. The great achievements in quality revolution in various industries have come from restructured and metamorphosed business processes. It is seen that healthcare and non-healthcare literature has an abundance of evidence to show the criticality of process management. Service process management essentially refers to the procedures, systems and technology that are required to streamline the service delivery. As noted from the revised Boynton and Victor Model for healthcare (McLaughlin and Kaluzny, 1999, p. 15) process enhancement requires that processes be analysed and modified to develop best practice approach using worker feedback and process-owning teams within the organization. For consistently delivering services, the key and support processes should be clearly analysed, understood, perfectly streamlined, standardized and simplified so that customers can receive the service without any difficulties. Nwabueze and Kanji (1997) analysed the implementation of TQM in the NHS of the UK and showed that process management in terms of identification of key processes, meeting patient needs and people ownership are critical to quality.

Healthcare services are unique in nature in that the delivery of clinical care involves a large variety of hospital staff (doctors, nurses, medical technologists, pharmacist, non-medical staff, etc.).

They all have varied backgrounds in terms of education and experience as well as service orientation toward patients. In addition, personal and professional preferences and information available to various groups of staff result in process variations (Huq, 1996). Therefore, process standardization ensures consistent delivery of services. Process management and improvement in healthcare services have shown a number of advantages such as improvements in overall turn around time, better patient satisfaction, cost minimization and savings, employee morale, reduction in waiting times, improved motivation of workers, patient safety, better patient outcomes, efficient resource utilization (Kohli et al., 1995; Anderson et al., 1996; Gonalez et al., 1997; Bharat et al., 1998; Klein et al., 1998; Moody et al., 1998; Poirier and Moran, 1998; Bharat et al., 1999; Singhal et al., 2001; Varghese, 2001; Chow-Chua and Goh, 2002; Reddy et al., 2002; Chang and Cheng, 2003; Reddy and Acharyulu, 2003; Murray, 2003). Studies have shown that the use of standard operating procedures and departmental protocol help standardize processes to minimize variations in healthcare services. Hospitals have a number core processes such as diagnostics, emergency services, trauma care, patient care, surgery, etc. as well as support processes including medical and non-medical processes such as laboratory services, medical records, ambulance, security, canteen, etc. Such processes have to be streamlined and integrated into providing high quality services so that patients not only get treated and feel healthy but are also getting those services in a timely manner without delays and are satisfied. In general, a number of process improvement techniques are available for improvement of processes from simple modification of the process to radical rethinking and revamping processes from scratch known as process re-engineering.

Tari (2005) concluded that customer-related issues and process management are the most important components of successful TQM implementation based on empirical research in 106 ISO firms in Spain. In an empirical study using hospital survey based on EQA model in Spain, the Netherlands and the UK, Kunst and Lemmink (2000) found that process management is an explanatory factor for high quality services followed by personnel management. Based on a case study of a hospital, Aghazadeh (2002) found that process focus and management was a critical factor for the implementation of TQM in the managed care industry in the US. Many quality award criteria include process management as crucial to overall quality (Flynn and Saladin, 2001; Meyer and Collier, 2001). From the above discussion, it is clear that process management is a critical factor validated in different sectors in order to achieve total quality. The identification of core and support processes is very essential and the processes need to be mapped and standardized, tracked on a regular basis and improvement should be achieved by regular monitoring and feedback.

6. Service Culture

Organizational culture is extremely important for improving the overall quality performance. Edgar Schein defined corporate culture as 'the basic assumptions driving life in a given organization' (Schein, 1985 cited in Gaucher and Coffey, 1993, p. 148). Every organization has a culture created by the shared beliefs, values, norms and expectations of the workforce. A TQM process can revitalize an organization and allow people to feel passionately about work. According to Gaucher and Coffey (1993, pp. 148–151), peak performance begins with commitment: to the team, to excellence and to changing the organization. 'A strong culture, with well-socialized members, improves organizational effectiveness because it facilitates the exchange of information and coordination of behavior' (Denison, 1990 cited in Gaucher and Coffey, 1993, p. 148). Jabnoun (2001) identified respect, responsibility and empathy as values driving continuous improvement and humbleness, trust, openness and cooperation as enabling factors. Such an organizational culture would further facilitate optimum interactions with patients, families and other customers in service organizations such as hospitals.

Customers in service organizations are separated by only a very thin layer from the employees in which physical and psychological closeness between them is so great that only an organizational culture that stresses service quality throughout the organization could establish the seamlessness in the service delivery (Sureshchandar et al., 2001b). This is so very true in the case of healthcare services. Parasuraman et al. (1988) have emphasized that with good service culture in place, an organization is more likely to offer a reliable, responsive, empathetic service to various groups of customers. The perceived service quality attributes, namely reliability, responsiveness, empathy and assurance included by Parashuraman and others have time and again shown to be major determinants in service delivery performance. In healthcare, for instance, responsiveness, empathy and assurance at all levels of service operations assumes the highest level of importance considering emotions such as anxieties and fears with which the patients and families approach medical and non-medical personnel for consultation. The service orientation is nothing new to healthcare but just that the features cannot be assumed to be present in sufficient amounts across all levels of staff. Also, in diverse workforce with a wide range of educational and attitudinal backgrounds, which is characteristic of healthcare services, explicitly stated cultural values and practice is essential. Service culture is actually the extent to which the employees at all levels realize that the real purpose of their existence is 'service to customers'. In general, customer focus and satisfaction is the goal of TQM and one important strategy to achieve would be through a strong internal service culture in an organization. Zabada et al. (1998) further emphasize a culture of heroism to commercial goals without losing the dignity of healthcare services as very important. Collins (1994) discussing the approaches to quality has emphasized that personal qualities based on Japanese wisdom (precepts) such as cooperation, patience, self-discipline and obligation are crucial. Importance of coordination and team work can be gauged by a quote from Jongi Noguchi: 'TQM is based on 100 men making one step, rather than one making 100 steps'.

As TQM practice further evolved, the importance of organizational culture as critical to total quality has been identified by many researchers. Black and Porter (1996) have emphasized a corporate culture committed to quality improvement as a critical factor in manufacturing. Employee involvement and empowerment in developing human resources for total quality achievement is available in the service sector literature. Research by Sureshchandar et al. (2001a, b) validated the 'Service Culture' factor as a critical factor. In a study by Huq (1996), activities to remove barriers to consensus for TQM approach and methods as well as proper communication of the values, attitudes and staff involvement figured as important strategies for establishing service culture in hospitals. Mandal et al. (2000) based on empirical observations of QM practices in the Indian manufacturing industry concluded that improvement of organizational culture including team work, harmony and participation are essential to quality improvement programmes. Similarly, Lakhe and Mohanty (1994) emphasized that TQM implementation in a developing country like India should focus on creating a total quality-oriented culture and commitment. Oakland (1997) stressed that creating culture or changing the culture in terms of people interactions, norms for working groups, values, rules of the game and the climate are essential to TQM practice. From the literature review analysis, *Service Culture* dimension for TQS would include the service orientation; open, trusting and good relationships instead of strong bureaucratic relations among employees of different levels; strong belief in providing high quality services; strong feelings toward work and the organization and working amicably in teams.

7. Servicescapes

Facility and service tangibles have been one of the most recognized factors in services only next to human interactions between customers (patients and families in healthcare primarily) and the service providers. The tangible facets of the service facility, i.e., the man-made physical environment such as equipment, machinery, signage and employee appearance – the 'servicescape', strongly influence both employees and customers in physiological, psychological, emotional, sociological and cognitive ways, particularly as the core service becomes more intangible (Sureshchandar et al., 2001a, p. 354). Such an impact of overall facility tangibles on perceived quality aspect of services is often highlighted in literature. The physical environment's influence on behaviours and image creation about the organization and its employees, particularly in services such as hotels, restaurants, professional offices, banks, retail stores and hospitals is well recognized in literaıure (Sureshchandar et al., 2001a). Works of Parasuaraman et al. (1985, 1988) and Zeithaml et al. (1990), which focused on conceptualizing quality performance in the service industry, identified facility tangibles as an important dimension of perceived service quality. In healthcare, the Servicescapes factor attains greater importance as it is closely connected to healing (impact of external environment) in terms of hygiene and feeling comfortable whether in waiting rooms or in wards. Movement of patients to and from various departments also needs appropriate planning for swiftness of transferring patients in emergencies or locating specific areas for further testing or consultation. For instance, Macdonald (1994) argued that the feature of quietness in the wards, cleanliness and well equipped with patient-oriented service as well as technical equipment is part of healthcare delivery process. Goonan (1995) highlights that features are defined as the aspects to patient care that attract patients that distinguish one practitioner from another or one hospital care from others, and facility tangibles are a part of such features. Visually appealing physical facilities, technology to ease/enhance customer-provider interactions and neatness of the surrounding emerged as significant factors in a study by Rodger et al. (1999) on quality performance of healthcare facilities. Perceptions definitely play a major role in physician, hospital and healthcare procedure or plan selection. In general, patients are viewed more as a source of perceptual than factual information about healthcare experience (Collingwood, 1996). Study by Bitner (1992) on the impact of physical surroundings on customers and employees showed that the Servicescapes not only attracted or deterred entry but also influence the degree of success of consumer experiences in accomplishing their plans once inside the facility. In fact, consumers look for cues in the surroundings about the firm's ability to deliver quality service even before an actual service delivery takes place and this would influence future experiences in the facility. In the healthcare context, Aggarwal and Zairi (1997) and Mohanty et al. (1996) have also highlighted the importance of facility tangibles.

Servicescapes, then can be viewed as 'a sum total of all possible moments of truth experienced by the customers-both human and non-human that provides the rationale behind the customers' perception of the service business and satisfaction they derive from it' (Sureshchandar et al., 2001b, p. 386). The facility tangibles apply more to service organizations and are not viewed as a critical factor in manufacturing. It includes ambient conditions such as temperature, ventilation, noise, odour, etc. Also, signs, signboards, symbols, advertisement boards, pamphlets, educational materials, employee appearance and other artefacts in the organization form an important part of Servicescapes. In a healthcare organization, physical layout of the premises, furnishings, ramps, lifts, etc. also have an impact not only perceptual factors but also in actual servicing of patients.

8. Administrative System

Hospitals are complex organizations wherein a number of medical and non-medical activities are set up, and issues like day-to-day functioning of the hospital operations, monitoring, governing, etc. need to be streamlined. It is very clear that different stakeholder groups interact and influence the functioning of a typical healthcare unit in unique ways. Four major stakeholder groups were identified as important by Kanji and SÁ (2003): Internal members (e.g., administrators and managers, doctors, nurses, paramedical, etc.); Suppliers (equipment, pharmaceutical, etc.); Customers and purchasers (patients, families, local communities, other practitioners/referral sources, insurance companies, etc.); and Regulators and others (government, health authorities, professional bodies, financial institutions, observers). Governance and administrative processes eventually determine the integration of various hospital activities. Healthcare organizations use a number of internal and external audits related to management of staff, patients and other stakeholders (Nwabueze and Kanji, 1997). Hospitals use various mechanisms to govern and integrate all activities. Clinical division and Support Directorates are essential and their overall performance is periodically assessed and reviewed. A number of committees, medical and non-medical related committees, are used to set standards and ensure the smooth running of the hospital activities. Activities such as billing, recovery, claims, waiving of fees, staff benefits, etc., need to be integrated and administrative processes are very essential to the overall performance. Further, interdepartmental coordination and monitoring is essential for ensuring that multiple stakeholder needs are met.

Lin and Clousing (1995) surveying the practices of TQM in healthcare found that multiple measures of quality demonstrated the complexity of the phenomenon and its unique evolution in the healthcare environment. The support mechanisms to ensure TQS included administrative support in actually implementing a number of management decisions. Activities such as reallocating resources, allotting time to work on TQM, supporting policy changes, holding department meetings, creating various steering teams and monitoring becomes essential. The administrator's role is charged with the responsibility of systematically and continually exploring the quality dynamics in the hospital. Mohanty et al. (1996) discussing the parameters relating to patient care and their subsequent measurement highlighted the importance of administrative factors and functions of different boards in a healthcare organization. Aggarwal and Zairi (1997) emphasized the role of administrative activities and processes as very important in TQM in order to streamline primary healthcare orientation in NHS in the UK.

Baldrige healthcare criteria have included administrative and business operations management as a sub-category under Patient Healthcare Design and Services (Meyer and Collier, 2001). From the studies, the following activities of administrative services are identified as crucial, namely streamlining of various administrative functions across the hospital and measuring the performance of administrative processes through feedback from different stakeholders, coordinating and monitoring activities of committees involved in quality and ensuring proper documentation from legal and regulatory aspects of healthcare services.

9. Measurement, Information and Analysis

Anything to be controlled or improved has to be measured. Measurement is a central element of any TQM effort. One of the slides quoted by Johnson and McLaughlin (1999, p. 93) used in a number of training programmes in CQI read: 'In God we trust, all others send data'. In healthcare, data are full of 'factoids', opinions and anecdotes masquerading as facts and as data. Using scientific approach requires data to evaluate the current situation, analyse and improve processes, and tract progress. For heathcare, measurement techniques can come from industrial models of quality management and those developed in the specialties of biostatistics, economics, epidemiology and health services research. The general model of Plan, Do, Check, Act (PDCA) cycle along with data and analytical tools are useful. A number of tools are available which are very useful for measurement and analysis of data so that meaningful information can be extracted for overall improvement of various processes across the healthcare facilities. Flow charts, cause-and-effect diagrams, check sheets, Pareto charts or diagrams, histograms, run charts, regression analysis, control charts, etc. are all used in healthcare (Gaucher and Coffey, 1993, pp. 319–96; Johnson and McLaughlin, 1999, pp. 93–128). In general, information measures the organization's scope, validity, use and management of data and information that underlie its overall quality system.

Quality Data Reporting, Internal Quality Information Usage, SPC Usage, Quality Improvement Measurement Systems, Quality Improvement Measurement Systems, Measures of Costs of Quality, Statistical Evidence of Quality, Evaluation, and Information and Analysis are the factors which correspond to measurement, information and analysis system. For healthcare, MBNQA includes Measurement, Analysis and Knowledge Management with sub-factors of Management of Information and Data, Performance Comparisons and Benchmarking, and Analysis and use of Organizational level-data (Meyer and Collier, 2001). In healthcare, the pioneers of quality such as Donabedien, Berwick, Bluementhal, Kazandjian, McLaughlin and Kaluzny have highlighted the importance of evidence-based medicine and measurement in healthcare. Scientification of the practice of medicine cannot be ignored anymore.

Reduction of variation, process improvements and internal benchmarking are some of the major applications of measurement and data analysis at the organizational level. Variation exists and always will in every process, more evident in medical processes and it has to be constantly reduced. Every patient is different and the processes used to treat individual patients will have to vary and this is an important characteristic of the healthcare environment. Two kinds of variations can be identified so that they can be controlled: First, common cause (also referred to as systemic and internal) is inherent in the processes, generally random in nature; second, special source which can be attributed to a particular source, is non-random in nature. Blumenthal (1994) goes on to say 'Only by becoming the masters of variation-by understanding it better than any other party to the healthcare debate – can they (physicians) regain the scientific credibility that will enable them to reclaim the high ground in shaping healthcare reform, thereby protecting their patients' interests and their own'. Benneyan et al. (2003) have further stressed that measurement of data from healthcare processes display a natural variation which can be modelled using a variety of statistical distributions. Use of control charts (tools of SPC), for instance, can often yield insights into data more quickly and easy to use for decision-making than traditional statistical methods, e.g., control charts for flash sterilization rate, laboratory turn around time, surgical site infection rates, appointment access satisfaction, infectious waste monitoring, etc. can be used to study variations and improvements after specific intervention techniques. Based on empirical research, Huq (1996) concluded that statistical evidence of quality is a critical dimension for TQM for hospitals.

Herbert et al. (2003) evaluated the use of quality control tools and statistical process control (SPC) in 37 service organizations including banks, hospitals, courier services and utilities in the UK.

Flow charts, histograms, check sheets and arrow diagrams were the most popular tools used in these organizations. The general benefits reported were:

- Improving consistency and process performance in service delivery
- Creating defect-free process and service
- Increasing productivity and reducing operating costs
- Promoting teamwork
- Improving communication between departments and employees
- Increasing organization's reputation and market share

The study indicated that the most important factors in making the QC tools and SPC work were management commitment, training and education, communication and teamwork, and cooperation.

In many companies, benchmarking is a key component of the TQM process. Profitability and growth flow from a clear understanding of how business is performing, not just against its previous accomplishment, but against the toughest competitors or world-class organizations (Ghobadian and Woo, 1996). Harrington (1997) reported that process benchmarking showed a high correlation to high performance of organization and that SPC did not have an impact on performance though it did not have a negative effect. Benchmarking in healthcare has been emphasized as an important factor for improving services (Aggarwal and Zairi, 1997).

Integrated and accessible information is a necessary ingredient for healthcare organizations for implementing quality management strategies. Almost all quality models have incorporated information and analysis as a critical factor. Rivers and Bae (1999) explored the history and current status of information systems in healthcare organizations. From an extensive literature review, they established that aligning information system for effective TQM implementation in healthcare organization is increasingly becoming important. Ang et al.'s (2000) empirical research on the impact of Information Technology on quality management in the Malaysian public-sector companies found that Information Technology had a significant effect on all the critical factors of TQM including leadership, strategic planning, output quality assurance, important innovations, information and analysis, HR utilization, customer satisfaction and quality results. West (2001) studying the performance of NHS of the UK found that good information system would drive change in healthcare.

The discussion clearly establishes that the construct Measurement, Information and Analysis is critical and would include the following dimensions: patient information and clinical data; business and administrative services, monitoring and review of information and long-term strategy formulation. These are some of the important areas of application of information systems for quality management in hospitals. The importance of Hospital Information System (HIS) is a highly recognized area for managers to improvise upon constantly. Its contribution to overall quality performance is underscored.

10. Supplier Quality Management

Supplier Quality Management including partnerships with suppliers measures the ability of the organization to develop mutually beneficial relationships built on trust, sharing of knowledge and integration. It is an important aspect of TQM since the materials and equipment purchased actually determine the quality of finished goods and services. Organizations which manufacture the highest quality products have purchasing departments that rank quality rather than cost minimization as their major objective (Garvin, 1983 cited in Zhang et al., 2000, p. 733). If organizations pursue good supplier quality management, they should establish long-term quality activities, have detailed information about supplier performance, give feedback on the performance of the supplier's products, provide clear specifications about organizational requirements and regard product/service quality as the most important factor for selecting suppliers. The suppliers' role is critical in many ways according to Ahire et al. (1996). First, the quality of incoming materials (including parts in manufacturing) from the supplier determines the level of inspection effort of a buyer organization. Second, the quality of the supplied materials determines the final product quality. Third, supplier's capability to react to a buyer firm's needs, in turn, can determine the buyer's flexibility in responding to customer needs (Ahire et al., 1996).

Criticality of Supplier Quality for TQS in healthcare is determined by the works of Huq (1996) and MBNQA (Meyer and Collier, 2001). In healthcare, a number of supplies go into actual provision of services including diagnostics and treatment procedures. Drugs, various equipments, surgical, medical supplies, hospital furniture, patient-care related, new technologies, etc. are essential to producing healthcare services. Timelines and availability along with quality materials directly influence the health outcomes and in turn patient outcomes, satisfaction and the patients' and families future relationships with the service provider. Huq (1996) has reported that supplier development, e.g., lab, radiology, EKG, medicines, hospital essentials, is also consequential to the quality of care provided by the hospitals. Though the analysis showed that certification of the suppliers have not been addressed by all the hospitals studied, successful ventures have been reported in moving to a just-in-time approach for much of the inventory. The supplier development was also found to be high on the average scores across the hospitals studied.

11. Customer Focus and Satisfaction

To achieve quality, it is essential to know what customers want and to provide products or services. Customer satisfaction is the ultimate goal of any TQM programme because organizations can outdo their competitors by effectively addressing customers' needs and demands, and anticipating and responding to their evolving interests and wants. A successful organization recognizes the need to put the customer first in every decision made. The key to quality management is maintaining a close relationship with the customer in order to fully determine the customer needs, as well as receive feedback on the extent to which those needs are being met. Customer satisfaction is a very important measure of the company's performance and helps predict the future success or failure of an organization. In order to enhance customer satisfaction, customer complaints should be treated with top priority (Zhang et al., 2000; Sureshchandar et al., 2001a). The competitive advantage in a quality revolution comes from customer delight and the management's responsibility is to ensure that that satisfaction manifests itself as commitment in the long run (Kanji and SÁ, 2003). Ang et al. (2000) validated the customer requirements determination, customer satisfaction evaluation and relationship management as dimensions of the critical factor of customer satisfaction.

From a typical marketing perspective, parties exchange goods and/or services from the context for dis/satisfaction measures. The expectancy disconfirmation model used to explain post-purchase satisfaction suggests that consumer satisfaction can be simply defined as '... the evaluation rendered that the experience was at least as good as it was supposed to be' (Hunt, 1977 cited in Savitz, 1999, pp. 129–30). Healthcare is a market and shares similarities with conventional markets. Quality and value are currently convergent concepts in healthcare. The importance of patients as customers has increased the focus on quality management and value delivery (Walters and Jones, 2001). The concept of customers in healthcare would include patients, their families, public, healthcare professionals, insurance companies, third party payers, etc. In fact, everyone is a supplier and a customer at different times (Gaucher and Coffey, 1993, pp. 32–36). The complexity of patient perceptions and attitudes together with sometimes limited cognitive ability to process the nature of their own healthcare situation serves to complicate the decision process beyond attributes of patients' immediate health concern. Expectations are also shaped by a variety of inputs such as personal experiences as well as those of family and friends, physician recommendations and direct advertising campaigns (Savitz, 1999, pp. 129–46). Further, the ultimate objective of the healthcare system is to improve health and not just treat sick patients. Therefore, a comprehensive analysis of health status and needs may lead to the ability to serve customers better and to improve the health of the community around (Gaucher and Coffey, 1993, pp. 32–36).

Increased global competition, where high quality and low cost are at premium, has led to a increased interest in continuous improvement (Jabnoun, 2001). In the UK, competition earlier was about consultant recruitment. As consumers switched to NHS from fee-paying services because of perceived improvements of NHS services, private providers of healthcare had to reorient to competitive market strategy with an emphasis on differentiation on quality. A sound understanding of the customers and their requirements is crucial in private healthcare (Holloway and Mobbs, 1994). Wensing and Elwyn (2003) have highlighted that increased participation of patients and public in healthcare is desirable. Considering patients' views can improve processes and outcomes as well as satisfaction. A number of methods are used such as questionnaires, focus groups and feedback surveys to study patients' preferences for care, evaluations of what occurred or factual reports of care. Such measures should be assessed for validity, preferably by rigorous qualitative studies. In fact, medical consumerism is on the rise and better-informed patient population and families demand high-quality services (Boyce, 1997). Research by Carman (2000) on patient perceptions of service quality showed that patients evaluated technical dimensions of nursing care, physician care and outcome as more important than the accommodation functions of the hospital care. Therefore, it is important to improve both the perceived (affective dimensions of service quality) as well as clinical aspects of care.

Consumer satisfaction provides a useful outcome measure of the quality of care offered. It has been reported from literature that some of the benefits of measuring patient/enrollee satisfaction include increased profitability, increased market share, improved patient retention, improved collections, increased patient referrals, improved patient compliance, continuity of care, reduced hospitalization and length of stay, increased willingness to recommend the organization to family and friends, and reduced risk of malpractice. Intercorrelations among satisfaction, quality and loyalty have been reported to be quite significant (Savitz, 1999, pp. 129–46).

From the above discussion, it is clear that customer focus and quality should be the driving force behind day-to-day operations and customer satisfaction, which is a crucial goal of TQS management of a healthcare organization. Accurately analysing customer needs, expectations, measuring and meeting those needs are essential. Complaints and grievances should be handled in appropriate manner so that service recovery can take place and causes of complaints should be minimized or eliminated in future operations.

12. Key Results

As managers implement long-term quality management techniques and gradually extend it to the whole organization, the importance of evaluating the key result areas becomes apparent as quality is used by most as a competitive strategy. The goal then of TQS would be superior customer orientation, satisfaction and overall business results. Harrington (1997) reported that improvements in performance such as profitability, productivity and quality are good indicators of a successful implementation of TQM. Ang et al. (2000) included product and service quality, productivity, waste reduction or elimination, employee satisfaction as items under 'Quality Results' criteria. Such key results have to be monitored on a regular basis to ensure that the organization is progressing well and that the quality management programmes have an impact. The MBNQA has included business results as a criterion and in fact has assigned more weights to the criteria over the years (Flynn and Saladin, 2001).

In healthcare, McLaughlin and Simpson (1999, pp. 34–56) have concluded that a continuous quality improvement programme can and will provide benefits such as profitability, employee satisfaction, reduced costs and improved patient survival, and continuity of care. It is reported that market gains such as hospital loyalty, reputation for quality, increased market share are possible with higher patient and physician satisfaction which eventually result in the hospitals' ability to charge higher prices. This when combined with reduced costs with better patient recovery and efficient process would give rise to higher profits. Based on an empirical survey research on market orientation, Kumar et al. (1997) found that survival and growth/profit emphasis were critical factors. Profitability of all units of a hospital and earning revenues were found to be very important to improve performance relative to competitors. Raju and Lonial's (2002) study based on the survey of top executives of the hospitals and path model analysis, found a linear relationship among the constructs 'quality and market environment', 'quality and market outcomes' and 'financial performance'. Chow-Chua and Goh (2002) have highlighted the importance of tracking progress of the hospital quality management programme with key performance indicators such as net income margin and customer loyalty/retention rates. In a case study of a large public hospital, they integrated the criteria of Singapore Quality Award criteria (for the implementation of quality programme) and Balanced Score Card indicators successfully so that the senior and middle managers can use the indicators developed to obtain a comprehensive glimpse of the organization's performance in meeting its quality, operational and financial goals. In a multi-country study of hospitals (Spain, the UK and the Netherlands) using the EQA model, Kunst and Lemmink (2000) concluded that though TQM was linked to business performance only to a limited degree, progress in TQM leads to higher business performance of the hospital, indicating the efficiency (cost effect), and to a higher perceived service quality by patients, indicating its effectiveness. Meyer and Collier's (2001) empirical research using Baldrige healthcare pilot criteria included organization performance results under patient care; support services; community health services; administrative, business and supplier results, and accreditation and assessment areas.

Quality is a self-improvement as well as a competitive strategy. Healthcare organizations like any other business enterprise have profit orientation even though the primary goal is patient care and saving lives. Overall patient care results and the success of the new services launched by the hospitals are naturally key result areas that the hospitals would be monitoring on a regular basis, especially so when quality is implemented as a competitive strategy. Profitability, cost minimization and financial viability of projects along with acquiring new patient groups as customers, reputation of the hospitals, employee performance and satisfaction are all important as indicators of the overall results of quality management.

13. Social Responsibility

The concept of corporate citizenship is very important for an organization to be successful, progress toward achieving business excellence and sustaining gains. In healthcare, this in fact can be considered inbuilt because of the nature of the service itself. A typical healthcare delivery system such as a hospital utilizes a number of resources (human, material and knowledge) which are used in a series of processes that ultimately aim to improve the medical condition of the patient and contribute to healthier communities (Rivers and Bae, 1999; Kanji and SÁ, 2003). Donabedian (1973, cited in Durán-Arenas, 1999, pp. 14–15) in his seminal work on healthcare quality has highlighted the importance of social contract that a physician works under – 'Physicians are responsible for the well-being of their patients as well as general well-being of society' – which is different from the one that regulates industrial work and business transactions. Therefore, in many organizations physicians face a demand to achieve equity in the distribution of the benefits of healthcare, while they face the need to reach a balance between cost, quality and access. It is therefore important for both healthcare providers (directly in touch with patients) as well as managers to have a social orientation.

Kazandjian (1999, pp. 270–272) has stressed that performance improvement has to be seen in the context of the environment in which the healthcare delivery system is situated. At the same time, the environment can also want the hospital to fulfil the organization's social mission. The organization needs to be socially accountable and be sensitive and change to the ever-renewed social expectations based upon values, economic imperatives and the information infusion. In order to be fully attuned to the community, a hospital board should be able to prove that it satisfies those needs. Good planning, good documentation and good analysis of local needs will always be good policy.

Public responsibility and citizenship has been found to be a sub-category of leadership in many TQM models with critical factors (Sila and Ebrahimpour, 2003). The EQA and MBNQA both have incorporated the social responsibility criteria in the models. The EQA model has incorporated 'effect on society' as part of results of TQM along with employee and customer satisfaction and business results. Kunst and Lemmink's (2000) empirical research on identifying success parameters of quality management and business performance based on the EQA model, factor 'effect on society' emerged as critical to the success of quality management. The social issues of interest for the organization were issues of environment, safety, well-being, employment and working conditions. Similarly, Meyer and Collier's (2001) research using Baldrige criteria in healthcare organizations included the 'Public Responsibility and Citizenship' as one of the dimensions of Leadership criterion using the following measuring scales: integration of public responsibility into performance improvement efforts; ethical behaviour of employees; improving community services and respond to community emergencies.

Social and community obligations become important to have a good image and grow, for any organization, much more so in healthcare. Social responsibility becomes indispensable for organizations including healthcare. According to Sureshchandar et al. (2001a), this subtle factor nonetheless powerful dimension sends strong signals toward improving the organization's image and goodwill, and consequently affecting the customers' overall satisfaction with the services and their loyalty to the organization. Treating customers with respect, openness and team spirit, positive work attitude and reasonable pricing strategies are found to be important for providing total quality services.

Based on the above discussion 'Social Responsibility' was categorized as a critical factor encompassing the issues of integration of business activities in order to achieve excellent performance, ethical behaviours of employees, responding to community emergencies and improvement of community health. Further, environmental health, pollution and health education activities are considered important.

APPENDIX E

List of Participating Hospitals (Alphabetical Order)

1. A.J. Hospital and Research Centre, Mangalore
2. Apollo, Vizag, Andhra Pradesh
3. Apollo Gleneagles Hospitals Limited, Kolkata
4. Apollo Hospital Enterprise Ltd., Chennai
5. Bangalore Institute of Oncology, Bangalore
6. Bhagawan Mahavir Jain Heart Centre, Bangalore
7. Bollineni Superspeciality Hospital, Nellore
8. Bombay Hospital & Medical Research Centre, Mumbai
9. Care Hospital, Nampally, Hyderabad
10. C.U. Shah Medical College, Surendranagar, Gujarat
11. Department of Atomic Energy Hospital, Kalpakkam
12. Dr T.M.A. Pai Hospital, Udupi
13. D.Y. Patil Hospital and Research Centre, New Mumbai
14. Father Muller Medical College Hospital, Mangalore
15. G. Kuppuswamy Naidu Memorial Hospital, Coimbatore
16. Hosmat Hospital, Bangalore
17. K.G. Hospital, Coimbatore
18. Kasturaba Medical College Hospital, Attavar, Mangalore
19. Leelavathi Hospital, Mumbai
20. Manipal Hospital, Bangalore
21. M.S. Ramaiah Hospital, Bangalore
22. M.H. Saboo Siddique Hospital, Mumbai
23. Max Hospital, Noida, UP
24. Moolchand Hospital, Delhi
25. M.V.J. Medical College, Bangalore
26. Narayana Hrudayalaya, Bangalore
27. NRI Medical College Hospital, Vijayawada
28. P.D. Hinduja National Hospital & Medical Research Centre, Mumbai

29. Sagar Apollo Hospital, Bangalore
30. Sankara Netralaya, Chennai
31. Santokba Durlabhji Memorial Hospital & Medical Research Institute, Jaipur
32. Sri Venkateswara Institute of Medical Sciences, Tirupathi
33. St. James Hospital, Chalakudy, Kerala
34. St. Johns Medical College Hospital, Bangalore
35. Sundar Hospital, Chennai
36. The Bangalore Hospital, Bangalore
37. The Madras Medical Mission, Chennai
38. Vydehi Institute of Medical Sciences and Research Centre, Bangalore
39. Yenepoya Medical College Hospital, Mangalore
40. Wockhardt Hospital & Heart Institute, Bangalore

References

Adinolfi, P. (2003) "Total quality management in public health care: A study of Italian and Irish hospitals", *Total Quality Management*, Vol. 14, No. 2, pp. 141–150.

Aggarwal, A.K. and M. Zairi (1997) "The role of total quality management in enabling a primary health-care orientation", *Total Quality Management*, Vol. 8, No. 6, pp. 347–359.

Aghazadeh, S.M. (2002) "Implementation of total quality management in the managed care industry", *The TQM Magazine*, Vol. 14, No. 2, pp. 79–91.

Ahire, S.L., D.Y. Golhar and M.A. Waller (1996) "Development and validation of TQM implementation constructs", *Decision Sciences*, Vol. 27, No. 1, pp. 23–56.

Andaleeb, S.S., N. Siddiqui and S. Khandakar (2007) "Doctors' service orientation in public, private and foreign hospitals", *International Journal of Health Care Quality Assurance*, Vol. 20, No. 3, pp. 253–263.

Anderson, D.J., R.G. Norton, G.E. Reed and J.W. Moran (1996) "Managing change: A tale of two hospitals in an integrated network", *The TQM Magazine*, Vol. 8, No. 3, pp. 27–34.

Ang, C., M. Davies and P.N. Finlay (2000) "Measures to assess the impact of information technology on quality management", *International Journal of Quality & Reliability Management*, Vol. 17, No. 1, pp. 42–65.

Applebaum, S.H. and L. Wohl (2000) "Transformation or change: Some prescriptions for health-care organizations", *Managing Service Quality*, Vol. 10, No. 5, pp. 279–298.

APVVP-Andhra Pradesh Vaidya Vidhana Parishad. "Health System Performance Assessment". Available at: http://health.ap.nic.in/apvvp/apvvpmap.htm and http://www. ihsnet.org.in/HealthSystemPerformanceAssessment/HPA.htm

Arya, S.K., D.K. Sharma, S.S. Nagarajan and V. Kaushal (2003) "Job redesigning: Key to cost containment and TQM in hospitals", *Journal of the Academy of Hospital Administrations*, Vol. 15, No. 1, pp. 39–41.

Bangalore Medical Directory (2005) Published by Universal Medifosys, Konena Agarhar, Bangalore.

Bedi, S., S. Arya and R.K. Sarma (2004) "Patient expectation survey: A relevant marketing tool for hospitals", *Journal of the Academy of Hospital Administrations*, Vol. 16, No. 1, pp. 15–24.

Beecham, L. (1999) "Government sets out vision for clinical governance", *BMJ* (News, 27 March), Vol. 318, p. 832.

Benneyan, J.C., R.C. Lloyd and P.E. Plsek (2003) "Statistical process control as a tool for research and healthcare improvement", *Quality & Safety in Health Care*, Vol. 12, pp. 458–464.

Berman, P. and P.R. Eliya (1993) "Government policies that influence the development of private provision", in *Factors Affecting the Development of Private Health Care Provision in Developing Countries*, Major Applied Research Paper No. 9, Health Financing & Sustainability (HFS) Project, Bethesda, USA.

Bharat, R. (1994) "Value engineering: A new concept in reducing cost of burn care", *Indian Journal of Plastic Surgery*, Vol. 27, pp. 86–89.

Bharat, V. (2001) "Excellence in health care: Overview of the experiences in Tata main hospital", *Health Administrator: The Official Journal of the Indian Society of Health Administrators*, Vols. 11–12, Nos. 1–2, pp. 1–3.

Bharat, V., B. Mohanty and N.K. Das (1999) "Waiting time reduction in outpatient services: An analogy to heart failure therapy", *Indian Journal of Occupational and Environmental Medicine*, Vol. 3, No. 4, pp. 181–184.

Bharat, V., S. Tripathy, A.K. Guha and A. Mitra (1998) "Fast track thrombolysis in acute myocardial infarction: A quality improvement project", *Indian Heart Journal*, Vol. 50, No. 2, pp. 167–171.

Bhardwaj, A., D.K. Sharma, R.K. Sarma and P.C. Chaubey (2001) "Expectations of people from quality health services in metropolitan city of Delhi and to propose a sound health care marketing strategy for private/corporate hospitals in Delhi", *Journal of the Academy of Hospital Administrations*, Vol. 13, No. 2, pp. 59–64.

Bhat, R. (1996) "Regulation of the private sector in India", *International Journal of Health Planning & Management*, Vol. 11, pp. 253–274.

Bitner, M.J. (1992) "Servicescapes: The impact of physical surroundings on customers and employees", *Journal of Marketing*, Vol. 56, No. 2, pp. 57–71.

Black, S.A. and L.J. Porter (1996) "Identification of the critical factors of TQM", *Decision Sciences*, Vol. 27, No. 1, pp. 1–21.

Blumenthal, D. (1994) "The variation phenomenon in 1994", *The New England Journal of Medicine*, Vol. 331, No. 15, pp. 1017–1018.

Boyce, N. (1997) "Quality in Australian health care: Moving the goalpost on a roughly paved road to improvement", in *The Effectiveness of CQI in Health Care: Stories from a Global Perspective*, V.A. Kazandjian (ed.), ASQC Health Care Series, Milwaukee, Wisconsin: ASQC Quality Press, pp. 109–113.

Brooks, A. and G. Zeitz (1999) "The effects of total quality management and perceived justice on organizational commitment of hospital nursing staff", *Journal of Quality Management*, Vol. 4, No. 1, pp. 69–93.

Brown, R.B. and L. Bell (1998) "Patient-centered audit: A user's quality model", *Managing Service Quality*, Vol. 8, No. 2, pp. 88–96.

Buchan, H. (1998) "Different Countries, different cultures: Convergent or divergent evolution of healthcare quality?", *Quality in Health Care*, Vol. 7 (Suppl): S62–S67. Available at: http://bmj.com/misc/qhc/62-67.shtml

Caldwell, C. (1997) "Accelerated improvement strategies in healthcare," paper given at the First Internatinal Conference on Managing Innovation in Public Services, Sheffield Hallan University, Sheffield, 2–3 April.

Carman, J.M. (2000) "Patient perceptions of service quality: Combining the dimensions", *Journal of Management in Medicine*, Vol. 14, No. 5/6, pp. 339–356.

Castle, N.G. (1999) "Quality improvement and top management in nursing homes", *Journal of Quality Management*, Vol. 4, No. 1, pp. 95–109.

CBHI-Central Bureau of Health Intelligence, Directorate of General Health Services, Ministry of Health & Family Welfare, Government of India, Cited on 9th July 2005. Available at: http://cbhidghs.nic.in/

Chanda, R. (2005) "The globalisation of healthcare services". Available at: http://www.financialexpress.com/columnists/full_column.php?content_id=93802

Chang, C. and B. Cheng (2003) "To establish a continuing care system of discharge planning by QFD", *TQM & Business Excellence*, Vol. 14, No. 8, pp. 903–918.

Chassin, M.R. and R.W. Galvin (1998) "The urgent need to improve health care quality", Consensus Statement, *JAMA*, September, Vol. 280, No. 11, pp. 1000–1005.

Chow-Chua, C. and M. Goh (2002) "Framework for evaluating performance and quality improvement", *Managing Service Quality*, Vol. 12, No. 1, pp. 54–66.

CII-McKinsey and Company (2002) *A report on healthcare in India: The road ahead.* CII and McKinsey, New Delhi.

Clarke, A. (2004) "Readmission to hospital: A measure of quality or outcome?", *Quality & Safety in Health Care*, Commentaries, Vol. 13, No. 1, pp. 10–11.

Coddington, D.C., L.E. Palmquist and W.V. Trollinger (1985) "Strategies for survival in the hospital industry", *Harvard Business Review*, Vol. 63, No. 3, pp. 129–138.

Collingwood, M.P. (1996) "Quality assurance versus the organizational goal: An NHS perspective", *Managing Service Quality*, Vol. 6, No. 6, pp. 21–24.

Collins, C.D., D.J. Hunter and A.T. Green (2000) "NHS reforms in the United Kingdom and learning from developing country experience", *Journal of Management in Medicine*, Vol. 14, No. 2, pp. 87–99.

Collins, P. (1994) "Approaches to quality", *The TQM Magazine*, Vol. 6, No. 3, pp. 39–43.

Counte, M.A. and S. Meurer (2001) "Issues in the assessment of continuous quality improvement implementation in health care organizations", *International Society for Quality in Health Care*, Vol. 13, No. 3, pp. 197–207.

Cuganeshan, S., G. Bradley and P. Booth (1997) "Service quality and organizational performance indicators", in *Managing Service Quality: Volume III of Series Quality Management in Services*, P. Kunst and J. Lemmink (eds.), Great Britain: Paul Chapman, pp. 161–181.

Cunha, M.P.E., J.V.D. Cunha and S. Dahab (2002) "Yin-yang: A dialectical approach to total quality management", *Total Quality Management*, Vol. 13, No. 6, pp. 843–853.

Das, N.K., S. Prasad and K. Jayaram (2001) "A TQM approach to implementation of handling and management of hospital waste in Tata main hospital", *Health Administrator: The Official Journal of the Indian Society of Health Administrators*, Vols. 11–12, Nos. 1–2, pp. 75–78.

DesHarnais, S.I. and C.P. McLaughlin (1999) "The outcome model of quality", in *Continuous Quality Improvement in Health Care: Theory, Implementation and Applications*, C.P. McLaughlin and A.D. Kaluzny (eds.), 2nd ed., Gaithersburg, MD: Aspen, pp. 57–92.

Dhanjal, H. (2001) "Quality circles: Tapping employee creativity", *Health Administrator: The Official Journal of the Indian Society of Health Administrators*, Vols. 11–12, Nos. 1–2, pp. 81–82.

Donaldson, L.J. and J.A.M. Gray (1998) "Clinical governance: A quality duty for health organizations", *Quality in Health Care*, Vol. 7 (Suppl): S37–S44. Available at: http://bmj.com/misc/qhc/37-44.shtml

Durán-Arenas L.D., J.D.M. Vallejo and R.S. Rodríquez (1997) "The Continuous Quality Improvement Program in the Mexican

Secretary of Health" In: The effectiveness of CQI in Health Care: Stories from a Global Perspective. Kazandjian V.A. (ed) ASQC Health Care Series. Milwaukee, Wisconsin: ASQC Quality Press; pp. 11–48.

Editor's choice, BMJ (2000) "Facing up to medical error". Available at: http://bmj.bmjjournals.com/cgi/content/full/320/7237/0

EFQM-European Foundation for Quality Management, Brussels, Belgium "The EFQM excellence model", Cited on 10th July 2005. Available at: http://www.efqm.org/Default.aspx? tabid=35

Eggli, Y. and P. Halfon (2003) "A conceptual framework for hospital quality management", *International Journal of Health Care Quality Assurance,* Vol. 16, No. 1, pp. 29–36.

Ennis, K. and D. Harrington (1999a) "Factors to consider in the implementation of quality within Irish health care", *Managing Service Quality*, Vol. 9, No. 5, pp. 320–326.

Ennis, K. and D. Harrington (1999b) "Quality management in Irish health care", *International Journal of Health Care Quality Assurance,* Vol. 12, No. 6, pp. 232–243.

Ernst and Young Healthcare (2003) Health care report 2003, prepared for Indian Healthcare Federation, New Delhi: Ernst & Young Pvt. Ltd., Secunderabad, India.

Flynn, B.B. and B. Saladin (2001) "Further evidence on the validity of the theoretical models underlying the Baldrige criteria", *Journal of Operations Management,* Vol. 19, No. 6, pp. 617–652.

Gaucher, E.J. and R.J. Coffey (1993) *Total Quality in Health Care: From Theory to Practice,* San Francisco: Jossey-Bass.

Ghobadian, A. and H.S. Woo (1996) "Characteristics, benefits and shortcomings of four major quality awards", *International Journal of Quality & Reliability Management,* Vol. 13, No. 2, pp. 10–44.

Ginter, P.M., L.E. Swayne and W.J. Duncan (2002) *Strategic Management of Health Care Organizations*, 4th ed., Malden, MA: Blackwell, pp. 1–49.

GoI-Government of India (2003) Ninth Five-Year Plan: 1997–2002, Government of India.

GoI-Government of India (2004) "Health sector reforms in India: Initiatives from nine states", August 2004, Bureau of

Planning, Directorate of General Health Services, Ministry of Health & Family Welfare, Government of India, New Delhi.

González C.J., González M. and Ríos N. (1997) "Improving the quality of service in an emergency room using simulation-animation and Total Quality Management" Computers and Industrial Engineering, Vol. 33, Nos. 1–2, pp. 97–100.

Goonan, K. Jennison (1995) *The Juran Prescription: Clinical Quality Management*, A Juran Institute Publication, San Francisco: Jossey-Bass.

Gumber, A. and V. Kulkarni (2000) "Health insurance for workers in the informal sector: Detailed results from a pilot study", NCAER, New Delhi, India.

Gupta, A. (1995) "Productivity measurement in service operations: A case study from the health-care environment", *Managing Service Quality*, Vol. 5, No. 5, pp. 31–35.

Gupta, A. (1998) "What and how of quality: A case study of Indraprastha Apollo hospital, New Delhi", IIHMR, Jaipur, PGD HHM Dissertation.

Gupta, S.K. (2004) "Quality dimensions in hospital infection control", *Express Healthcare Management*, 16th to 30th June 2004. Available at: http://www.expresshealthcaremgmt.com/20040630/criticaremgmt04.shtml

Gupta, S.K. and S. Kant (2002) "Quality dimension in hospital infection control" Journal of Academy of Hospital Administration, Vol. 14. No. 1. Available at http://www.indmedica.com/journals.php?journalid=6&issueid=21&articleid=182&action=article

Gyani, G.J. and M.B. Mittal (2001) "Application of ISO 9001: 2000 to health sector", JIIQM, *Indian Institute of Quality Management*, Jaipur, pp. 7–15.

Haigh, D. (2000) "Mergers in action: An examination of the efficacy of a merger between three NHS hospital trusts and the subsequent effects of that merger", *Total Quality Management*, Vol. 11, Nos. 4–6, pp. S589–S595.

Hair, J.F., Jr., Anderson, R.E., Tatham, R.L. and Black, W.C. (1995) Multivariate Data Analysis, 3rd ed, Macmillan Publishing Company, New York.

Harrington, H.J. (1995) "The new model for improvement: Total improvement management", *Business Process Re-engineering & Management Journal*, Vol. 1, No. 1, pp. 31–43.

Harrington, H.J. (1997) "The fallacy of universal best practices", *The TQM Magazine*, Vol. 9, No. 1, pp. 61–75.

Harte, H. and G. Etchart (1997) "Quality and Charge in the Provision of Health Care: The Relationship between Chaos and Quality. The Case Study of a Seattle Clinic" In: Managing Service Quality-Volume III of Series Quality Management in Services. Kunst P., & Lemmink J. (eds) Great Britain: Paul Chapman Publishing Ltd. pp. 149–60.

Harteloh, P.P.M. (2003) "Quality systems in health care: A sociotechnical approach", *Health Policy*, Vol. 64, No. 3, pp. 391–398.

Health Information of India & Directory of Hospitals in India, CBHI, Department of Health, Cited on 19th July 2005. Available at: http://www.cbhidghs.nic.in

Herbert, D., A. Curry and L. Angel (2003) "Use of quality tools and techniques in services", *The Service Industry Journal*, Vol. 23, No. 4, pp. 61–80.

Hewison, A. (2003) "Qualitative management research in the NHS: A classic case of counting to one?", *Journal of Health Organization & Management*, Vol. 17, No. 2, pp. 122–137.

Hind, M. (1996) "Are the cultures required to attain ISO 9000 and total quality management mutually exclusive?", *Training for Quality*, Vol. 4, No. 2, pp. 25–29.

Ho, W. (1999) "Organizational transformation for service excellence in a public hospital in Hong Kong", *Managing Service Quality*, Vol. 9, No. 6, pp. 383–388.

Holloway, B. and D. Mobbs (1994) "Customer focus groups: Developments in health care", *The TQM Magazine*, Vol. 6, No. 1, pp. 13–17.

Houghton, G. and D. Wall (2000) "Twelve tips on teaching about clinical governance", *Medical Teacher*, Vol. 22, No. 2, pp. 145–153.

Hurst, K. (1997) "The nature and value of small and community hospital accreditation", *International Journal of Health Care Quality Assurance*, Vol. 10, No. 3, pp. 94–106.

Huq, Z. (1996) "A TQM evaluation framework for hospitals: Observations from a study", *International Journal of Quality & Reliability Management*, Vol. 13, No. 6, pp. 59–76.

IBEF (2005) *India Brand Equity Foundation: Health Care*. Available at: http://www.ibcf.org/industry/healthcare.aspx

IBEF (2006) *India Brand Equity Foundation: Economy Services*. Available at: http://www.ibef.org/economy/services.aspx

IRDA Bill-Insurance Regulatory & Development Authority Bill, Cited on 19th September 2005. Available at: http://www.insuremagic.com/content/Agents/IRDAUpdate/irda_bill/main_ index.asp & http://www.irdaindia.org/

Jabnoun, N. (2001) "Values underlying continuous improvement", *The TQM Magazine*, Vol. 13, No. 6, pp. 381–387.

Jackson, S. (2001) "Successfully implementing total quality management tools within health care: What are the key actions?", *International Journal of Health Care Quality Assurance*, Vol. 14, No. 4, pp. 157–163.

Jain, K. (2004) "Debt trap: Stuck in a private hospital, more than 40 per cent of the hospitalized borrow money, sell their assets", *The Times of India*, Saturday, 20th November 2004, p. 7. Available at: http:/www.expresshealthcaremgmt.com/200220430/cover1.shtml

Jain, S.K. and G. Gupta (2004) "Measuring service quality: SERVQUAL vs. SERVPERF scales", *Vikalpa*, Vol. 29, No. 2, pp. 25–37.

JCAHO-Joint Commission on Accreditation of Healthcare Organizations, Cited on 12th September 2005. Available at: http://www.jointcommission.org/

Jesani, A. (1996) *Laws and Health Care Providers*, Mumbai: Centre for Enquiry into Health & Allied Themes.

Johnson, S.P. and C.P. McLaughlin (1999) "Measurement and statistical analysis in CQI", in *Continuous Quality Improvement in Health Care: Theory, Implementation and Applications*, C.P. McLaughlin and A.D. Kaluzny (eds.), 2nd ed., Gaithersburg, MD: Aspen, pp. 93–128.

Kandampully, J. and L. Butler (2001) "Service guarantees: A strategic mechanism to minimize customers' perceived risk in service organisations", *Managing Service Quality*, Vol. 11, No. 2, pp. 112–121.

Kanji, G.K. and P.M.E. SÁ (2003) "Sustaining healthcare excellence through performance measurement", *Total Quality Management*, Vol. 14, No. 3, pp. 269–289.

Kaulio, M.A. (1998) "Customer, consumer and user involvement in product development: A framework and a review of selected methods", Total *Quality Management*, Vol. 9, No. 1, pp. 141–149.

Kazandjian, V.A. (1997a) "From mythology to epidemiology: The Historic roots of continuous quality improvement", Introduction, in *The Effectiveness of CQI in Health Care: Stories from a Global Perspective*, V.A. Kazandjian (ed.), ASQC Health Care Series, Milwaukee, Wisconsin: ASQC Quality Press, pp. 1–9.

Kazandjian, V.A. (1997b) "Hoc opus, hic labor est", in *The Effectiveness of CQI in Health Care: Stories from a Global Perspective*, V.A. Kazandjian (ed.), ASQC Health Care Series, Milwaukee, Wisconsin: ASQC Quality Press, pp. 267–272.

Kazandjian, V.A. (2004) "Does appropriate prescribing result in safer care?", *Quality & Safety in Health Care*, Commentaries, Vol. 13, No. 1, pp. 9–10.

Khoo, H.H. and K.C. Tan (2003) "Managing for quality in the USA and Japan: Differences between the MBNQA, DP and JQA", *The TQM Magazine*, Vol. 15, No. 1, pp. 14–24.

Klein, D., J. Motwani and B. Cole (1998) "Quality improvement efforts at St. Mary's hospital: A case study", *Managing Service Quality*, Vol. 8, No. 4, pp. 235–240.

Köeck, C.M. (1997) "Doing better: A Global Medical Interest", Foreword xvii–xxiii, in *The Effectiveness of CQI in Health Care: Stories from a Global Perspective*, V.A. Kazandjian (ed.), ASQC Health Care Series, Milwaukee, Wisconsin: ASQC Quality Press.

Kohli, R., B. Kerns and G.A. Forgionne (1995) "The application of TQM in a hospital's casualty and pathology departments", *International Journal of Quality & Reliability Management*, Vol. 12, No. 9, pp. 57–75.

Krüger, V. (2001) "Main schools of TQM: The big five", *The TQM Magazine*, Vol. 13, No. 3, pp. 146–155.

Kumar, K., R. Subramanian and C. Yauger (1997) "Performance-oriented: Toward a successful strategy", *Marketing Health Services*, Vol. 17, No. 2, pp. 10–20.

Kunst, P. and J. Lemmink (2000) "Quality management and business performance in hospitals: A search for success parameters", *Total Quality Management*, Vol. 11, No. 8, pp. 1123–1133.

Lakhe, R.R. and R.P. Mohanty (1994) "Total quality management: Concepts, evolution and acceptability in developing countries", *International Journal of Quality & Reliability Management*, Vol. 11, No. 9, pp. 9–33.

Leatherman, S. and K. Sutherland (1998) "Evolving quality in the new NHS: Policy, process and pragmatic considerations", *Quality in Health Care*, Vol. 7 (Suppl): S54–S61. Available at: http://bmj.com/misc/qhc/54-61.shtml

Lin, B. and J. Clousing (1995) "Total quality management in health care: A survey of current practices", *Total Quality Management*, Vol. 6, No. 1, pp. 69–78.

Lindberg, E. (2002) "Managing complexity: Acknowledge the attraction patterns by making sense making and allowing the quality system to serve as the panoptic system", *International Journal for Health Care Quality Assurance*, Vol. 15, No. 5, pp. 213–217.

Logothetis, N. (2003) *Managing for Total Quality: From Deming to Taguchi and SPC*, New Delhi: Prentice Hall.

Low, S.P. (1998) "Managing Total Service Quality: A Systemic View" *Managing Service Quality*, Vol. 8, No. 1, pp. 34–45.

Lozano, A.R.P. (1997) "ISO 9000 and the total quality management models", *Library Management*, Vol. 18, No. 3, pp. 148–150.

Macdonald, J. (1994) "Services is Different", *The TQM Magazine*, Vol. 6, No. 1, pp. 5–7.

Macdonald, J. (1995) "Quality improvement in the NHS", *Managing Service Quality*, Vol. 5, No. 3, pp. 20–22.

Magd, H. and A. Curry (2003) "ISO 9000 and TQM: Are they complementary or contradictory to each other?", *The TQM Magazine*, Vol. 15, No. 4, pp. 244–256.

Mahapatra, P., S. Sinatra and P. Sridhar (2001) "A patient satisfaction survey in public hospitals", *Journal of the Academy of Hospital Administrations*, Vol. 13, No. 2, pp. 11–15.

Mandal, P., P.E.D. Love, A.S. Sohal and B. Bhadury (2000) "The propagation of quality management concepts in Indian manufacturing industry: Some empirical observations", *The TQM Magazine*, Vol. 12, No. 3, pp. 205–213.

Manjunath, U., A.K. Bhat and N.V.M. Rao (2007) "Content validation of total quality service constructs for hospitals: Observations from a study", Paper Accepted for presentation in The 10th International Conference Society for Global Business & Economic Development (SGBED) "Creativity and innovation: Imperatives for global business and development", Kyoto, Japan, August 8–11.

Manjunath, U. (2008). "Core issues in defining healthcare quality" *The ICFAI University Journal of Services Marketing*, Vol. VI, No. 4, December, pp. 72–78.

Manjunath, U. (2010) "Relationships among quality constructs for total quality services management in hospitals in India", *AIMS International Journal of Management*, Vol. 4, No. 2, pp. 77–92.

Mathews, B. and M.C. Clark (1997) "Quality determinants: The relationship between internal and external services", in *Managing Service Quality: Volume III of Series Quality Management in Services*, P. Kunst and J. Lemmink (eds.), Great Britain: Paul Chapman, pp. 11–34.

MBNQA-Malcolm Balridge National Quality Program (2003) "Health care criteria for performance excellence", National Institute of Science & Technology. Available at: http://www.quality.nist.gov

McLaughlin, C.P. and A.D. Kaluzny (1999) "Defining quality improvement: Past, present and future", in *Continuous Quality Improvement in Health Care: Theory, Implementation and Applications*, C.P. McLaughlin and A.D. Kaluzny (eds.), 2nd ed., Gaithersburg, MD: Aspen, pp. 3–30.

McLaughlin, C.P. and K.N. Simpson (1999) "Does TQM/CQI work in health care?", in *Continuous Quality Improvement in Health Care: Theory, Implementation and Applications*, C.P. McLaughlin and A.D. Kaluzny (eds.), 2nd ed., Gaithersburg, MD: Aspen, pp. 34–56.

Meyer, S.M. and D.A. Collier (2001) "An empirical test of the causal relationships in the Baldrige Health Care Pilot Criteria", *Journal of Operations Management*, Vol. 19, No. 4, pp. 403–425.

MHSDP – Data Validation & Hospital Performance Analysis, Institute of Health Systems, Mission & Goals: Groom skills, gather evidence & generate knowledge for people's health. To improve efficacy, quality & equity of health systems, Cited on 15th July 2005. Available at: http://www.ihsnet.org.in/HealthSystemPerformanceAssessment/MHSDP.htm & http://www.expres shealthcaremgmt.com/20030215/hospi2.shtml

Mishra, M., T.B.K. Sinha, S.P. Bandhyopadhyay, A.K. Sarkar and S.C. Chawla (2001) "Indigenous substitute for optical system of imported microscopes through value engineering", *Health Administrator: The Official Journal of the Indian Society of Health Administrators*, Vols. 11–12, Nos. 1–2, pp. 63–67.

Mitra, S. (2001) "Benefits of total quality management in Tata main hospital", *Health Administrator: The Official Journal of the Indian Society of Health Administrators*, Vols. 11–12, Nos. 1–2, pp. 83–93.

Mohanty, R.P. and R.R. Lakhe (2006) *TQM in the Service Sector*, Mumbai: Jaico.

Mohanty, R.P., K. Santi and C. Haripriya (1996) "A model for evaluating TQM effectiveness in health-care systems", *Work Study*, Vol. 45, No. 2, pp. 14–17.

Moody, D., J. Motwani and A. Kumar (1998) "Implementing quality initiatives in the human resources department of a hospital: A case study", *Managing Service Quality*, Vol. 8, No. 5, pp. 320–326.

Motwani, J. (2001) "Critical factors and performance measures of TQM", *The TQM Magazine*, Vol. 13, No. 4, pp. 292–300.

Mukherjee, A. (2005) "Regular tests for doctors? Health Ministry prescribes fresh exams every five years", *The Times of India*, New Delhi, Thursday, March 17th, p. 1.

Murray, P. (2003) "Applying quality management tools to medical photography services: A pilot project", *Journal of Audiovisual Media in Medicine*, Vol. 26, No. 1, pp. 23–26.

NABL, Department of Science & Technology, India. Cited on 19th August 2005. Available at: http://www. nabl.india.org/

Naidu, A. (2009) "Factors affecting patient satisfaction and health care quality", *International Journal of Health Care Quality Assurance*, Vol. 22, No. 4, pp. 366–318.

Nandraj, S. (1994) "Beyond law and the Lord: Quality of private health care", *Economic & Political Weekly*, Vol. 29, No. 27, pp. 1680–1685.

Nandraj, S. and R. Duggal (1996) *Physical Standards in the Private Health Sector: A Case Study of Rural Maharashtra*, Mumbai: Centre for Enquiry into Health & Allied Themes.

Nandraj, S., A. Khot and S. Menon (1999) *Accreditation of Hospitals: Breaking Boundaries in Health Care*, Mumbai: Centre for Enquiry into Health & Allied Themes.

Nandaraj, S., A. Khot, S. Menon and R. Brugha (2001) "A stakeholder approach towards accreditation", *Health Policy and Planning*, Vol. 16 (Suppl 2): 70–79.

Nandraj, S., N. Madhiwala, R. Sinha and A. Jesani (1998) *Women and Health Care in Mumbai: A Study of Morbidity, Utilisation and Expenditure on Health Care in the Metropolis*, Mumbai: Centre for Enquiry into Health & Allied Themes.

Narang, R. (2010) "Measuring perceived quality in healthcare services in India", *International Journal of Health Care Quality Assurance*, Vol. 23, No. 2, pp. 171–186.

National Family Health Survey (NFHS–2) The National Family Health Survey–2 India 1998–1999, International Institute for Population Sciences, IIPS & ORC Macro, 2000, IIPS: Mumbai. Available at: http://www.nfhsindia.org

Newman, K. (1997) "Re-engineering for service quality: The case of Leicester Royal Infirmary", *Total Quality Management*, Vol. 8, No. 5, pp. 255–264.

NHP-National Health Policy (2002) Ministry of Health & Family Welfare, Government of India. New Delhi. Available at http://mohfw.nic.in/NRHM/Documents/National_Health_Policy_2002.pdf

NIST-National Institute of Standards and Technology. Cited on 9th August 2005. Available at: http://www.nist.gov/

NSS-National Sample Survey, National Sample Survey Organization (1998) Morbidity & Treatment of Ailments, NSS 52nd round, July 1995–June 1996.

Nunnaly, J.C. (1988) *Psychometric Theory*, Englewood Cliffs, New Jersey: McGraw Hill.

Nwabueze, U. and G.K. Kanji (1997) "The implementation of total quality management in the NHS: How to avoid failure?", *Total Quality Management*, Vol. 8, No. 5, pp. 265–280.

Oakland, J.S. (1997) "Interdependence and cooperation: The essentials of total quality management", *Total Quality Management*, Vol. 8, Nos. 2–3, pp. S31–S35.

O'Keeffe, M. and D. O'Sullivan (1997) "Service Quality in the Irish Health Service" Total Quality Management, Vol. 8, No. 5, pp. 293–303.

Øvretveit, J. (1997) "A comparison of hospital quality programmes: Lessons for other services", *International Journal of Service Industry Management*, Vol. 8, No. 3, pp. 220–235.

Øvretveit, J. and D. Gustafson (2003) "Using research to inform quality programmes", *BMJ*, Vol. 326, pp. 759–761.

Parasuraman, A., V.A. Zeithaml and L.L. Berry (1985) "A conceptual model of service quality and its implication for further research", *Journal of Marketing*, Vol. 49, No. 4, pp. 41–50.

Parasuraman, A., V.A. Zeithaml and L.L. Berry (1988) "SERVQUAL: A multiple-item scale for measuring consumer perceptions of service quality", *Journal of Retailing*, Vol. 64, No. 1, pp. 12–40.

Phadke, A. (1993) *The Private Sector in Health Care in India*, Bombay: Foundation for Research in Community Health.

PHDCCI Analysis (2004) "India set to record high growth in medical tourism: PHDCCI", *The Hindu*, Saturday, June 26, New Delhi, p. 3.

Poirier, E.A. and J.W. Moran (1998) "Design for change in home health agency", *Managing Service Quality*, Vol. 8, No. 1, pp. 19–23.

Potter, C., P. Morgan and A. Thomson (1994) "Continuous quality improvement in an acute hospital: A report on an action research project in three hospital departments", *International Journal of Health Care Quality Assurance*, Vol. 7, No. 1, pp. 4–29.

Priebe, S. (2000) "Ensuring and improving quality in community mental health care", *International Review of Psychiatry*, Vol. 12, No. 3, pp. 226–232.

Rabbani, F., S.M. Wasim Jafri, F. Abbas, F. Jahan, N. Syed, G. Pappas, S.I. Azam, M. Brommels and G. Tomson (2009) "Culture and quality care perspectives in a Pakistani hospital", *International Journal of Health Care Quality Assurance*, Vol. 22, No. 5, pp. 496–513.

Raja, M.P.N., S.G. Deshmukh and S. Wadhwa (2007) "Quality award dimensions: A strategic instrument for measuring health service quality", *International Journal of Health Care Quality Assurance*, Vol. 20, No. 5, pp. 363–378.

Raju, P.S. and S.C. Lonial (2002) "The impact of service quality and marketing on financial performance in the hospital industry: An empirical examination", *Journal of Retailing & Consumer Services*, Vol. 9, No. 6, pp. 335–348.

Ramani, K.V. and D. Mavalankar (2005) Health System in India: Opportunities & Challenges, Working Paper No. 2005–07.03, Indian Institute of Management, Ahmedabad, India. Available at: http://www.iimahd.ernet.in/publications/data/2005-07-03 ramani.pdf

Rameshan, P. and S. Singh (2004) "Quality of service of primary health centres: Insights from a field study", *Vikalpa*, Vol. 29, No. 3, pp. 71–82.

Rao, A.T. and A.K. Agarwal (2003) "Medical errors and patient safety", *Journal of the Academy of Hospital Administrations*, Vol. 15, No. 1, pp. 15–21.

Ray, B. (1999) "Value engineering: A practical approach to managing cost in critical care", (Editorial) *Indian Journal of Critical Care Medicine*, Vol. 3, No. 1, pp. 4–8.

Ray, B. (2001) "Human resource planning in health care", *Health Administrator: The Official Journal of the Indian Society of Health Administrators*, Vols. 11–12, Nos. 1–2, pp. 14–16.

Reddy, B.K. and G.V.R.K. Acharyulu (2003) "A study on emergency care and patient discharge process: Application of network analysis", *Journal of the Academy of Hospital Administrations*, Vol. 15, No. 1, pp. 23–27.

Reddy, B.K., M. Arundhathy and G.V.R.K. Acharyulu (2002) "A strategy for successful TQM in a corporate hospital: A study using six sigma", *Journal of the Academy of Hospital Administrations*, Vol. 14, No. 2, pp. 7–14.

Reichheld, F.F. and W.E. Sasser (1990) "Zero-defection: Quality comes to services", *Harvard Business Review*, Vol. 68, No. 5, September–October, pp. 105–111.

Reserve Bank of India: An Analysis of India's Service Sector, Studies by Reserve Bank of India. Available at: http://www.indiaonestop.com/serviceindustry.htm

Ritchie, L. (2002) "Driving quality: Clinical governance in the National Health Service", *Managing Service Quality*, Vol. 12, No. 2, pp. 117–128.

Rivers, P.A. and S. Bae (1999) "Aligning information systems for effective total quality management implementation in health care organizations", *Total Quality Management*, Vol. 10, No. 2, pp. 281–289.

RKS (2003) "Rogi Kalyan Samithi: An innovative project for the management of public hospitals through community participation in the state of Madhya Pradesh". Available at: http://www.mp.nic.in/health/mths.pdf

Rodger, J.A., P.G. Pendharkar and D.J. Paper (1999) "Management of information technology and quality performance in health care facilities", *International Journal of Applied Quality Management*, Vol. 2, No. 2, pp. 251–269.

Ruyter, K.D. and M. Wetzels (1996) "Two sides of the same story: Measuring different quality perceptions of the dyadic service encounter with the SERVCON instrument", *Total Quality Management*, Vol. 7, No. 6, pp. 595–603.

Sahni, A. (2001) "Introduction", *Health Administrator: The Official Journal of the Indian Society of Health Administrators*, Vols. 11–12, Nos. 1–2, pp. 1–4.

Samaddar, D.P., S. Kumar, A. Sunder, B. Ray, A. Ahmed, S. Sreedevi and P.K. Sahu (2001) "Value engineering in Tata main hospital ICU", *Health Administrator: The Official Journal of the Indian Society of Health Administrators*, Vols. 11–12, Nos. 1–2, pp. 45–58.

Saraph, J.V., P.G. Benson and R.G. Schroeder (1989) "An instrument for measuring the critical factors of quality management", *Decision Sciences*, Vol. 20, No. 4, pp. 810–829.

Savitz, L.A. (1999) "Measuring consumer satisfaction", in *Continuous Quality Improvement in Health Care: Theory, Implementation and Applications*, C.P. McLaughlin and A.D. Kaluzny (eds.), 2nd ed., Gaithersburg, MD: Aspen, pp. 129–146.

Shaw, C.D. (2000) "External quality mechanisms for health care: Summary of the ExPeRT project on visitatie, accreditation, EFQM and ISO assessment of European Union countries", *International Journal for Quality in Health Care*, Vol. 12, No. 3, pp. 169–175.

Short, P.J. and M.A. Rahim (1995) "Total quality management in hospitals", *Total Quality Management*, Vol. 6, No. 3, pp. 255–263.

Shortell, S.M., J.L. O'Brien, J.M. Carman et al. (1995) "Assessing the Impact of Continuous Quality Improvement/Total Quality Management: Concept versus Implementation," Health Services Research, Vol. 30, No. 2, June 1995, pp. 377–401.

Sila, I. and M. Ebrahimpour (2003) "Examination and comparison of the critical factors of total quality management (TQM) across countries", *International Journal of Production Research*, Vol. 41, No. 2, pp. 235–268.

Silvestro, R. (2001) "Towards a contingency theory of TQM in services: How implementation varies on the basis of volume and variety?", *International Journal of Quality & Reliability Management*, Vol. 18, No. 3, pp. 254–288.

Singh, S. and A. Mukherjee (2004) "India hits rock bottom on public health spending and only one doctor for 1800 people", *The Times of India*, Thursday, July 29, New Delhi, pp. 1–6.

Singhal, S., R. Tata, M. Kar, R. Sinha, S. Trivedi and G. Jaganath (2000) "Reduction of perinatal mortality rate in Tata main hospital: A quality improvement project", *The Journal of Obstetrics & Gynecology of India*, Vol. 50, No. 6, pp. 54–58.

Srivastava, N. (2003) "Experts call for quality standards to boost medical tourism", *Express Healthcare Management*, 16th to 30th June. Available at http://www.expresshealthcaremgmt.com/20030630/focus1.shtml

Statistical Outline of India (2001–2002) Tata Services Limited, Mumbai.

Sureshchandar, G.S., C. Rajendran and R.N. Anantharaman (2001a) "A conceptual model for total quality management in service organizations", *Total Quality Management*, Vol. 12, No. 3, pp. 343–363.

Sureshchandar, G.S., C. Rajendran and R.N. Anantharaman (2001b) "A holistic model for total quality services", *International Journal of Service Industry Management*, Vol. 12, No. 4, pp. 378–412.

Sutcliffe, K.M. (2004) "Defining and classifying medical error", *Quality & Safety in Health Care*, Commentaries, Vol. 13, No. 1, pp. 8–9.

Sutherland, K. and S. Dawson (1998) "Power and quality improvement in the new NHS: The roles of doctors and managers", *Quality in Health Care*, Vol. 7 (Suppl): S16–S23. Available at: http://bmj.com/misc/qhc/16-23.shtml

Tabish, S.A. (1998) "Towards development of professional management in Indian hospitals", *Journal of Management in Medicine*, Vol. 12, No. 2, pp. 109–199.

Tan, K.C. (2002) "A comparative study of 16 National quality awards", *The TQM Magazine*, Vol. 14, No. 3, pp. 165–171.

Tarí, J.J. (2005) "Components of successful total quality management", *The TQM Magazine*, Vol. 17, No. 2, pp. 182–194.

Tata Business Excellence Model (TBEM) in Mitra, S. (2001) "An introduction to Tata business excellence model", *Health Administrator: The Official Journal of the Indian Society of Health Administrators*, Vols. 11–12, Nos. 1–2, pp. 9–13.

The Hindu (2005) "Railway hospitals come under the purview of consumer courts: Indian Systems to be included in medical curriculum", *The Hindu*, New Delhi, Wednesday, 31st Jan, p. 3.

The Hindu (2006) "NHRC demands reply from AIIMS on hiked charges", *The Hindu*, Saturday, 7th Jan, p. 3.

Theodorakioglou, Y.D. and G.D. Tsiotras (2000) "The need for the introduction of quality management into Greek health care", *Total Quality Management*, Vol. 11, No. 8, pp. 1153–1165.

Thomson, R.G. and K. Hodgson (1997) "Quality in the British National health service", in *The effectiveness of CQI in Health Care: Stories from a Global Perspective*, V.A. Kazandjian (ed.), ASQC Health Care Series, Milwaukee, Wisconsin: ASQC Quality Press, pp. 135–192.

TNMSC (2003) Tamil Nadu Medical Services Corporation Limited, 10th Annual Report, 2003–2004.

U.S. Congress of Technology Assessment (1988) Cited in DesHarnais, S.I., P. Curtis and C.P. McLaughlin (1999) "The outcome model of quality", in *Continuous Quality Improvement in Health Care: Theory, Implementation and Applications*, C.P. McLaughlin and A.D. Kaluzny (eds.), 2nd ed., Gaithersburg, MD: Aspen, pp. 34–56.

Varghese, R. (2001) "Process reengineering in the radiology department in a corporate hospital", *Journal of the Academy of Hospital Administrations*, Vol. 13, No. 1, pp. 21–29.

Verma, D.P.S. and R. Sobti (2002) "Patient's perceptions of medical services", *Journal of Services Research*, Vol. 2, No. 1, pp. 123–134.

Victor, B. and A.C. Boynton (1998) Invented here: Maximizing your organisation's internal growth and profitability", Harvard Business School Press, Boston.

Vij, A., S.N. Williamson and S. Gupta (2001) "Knowledge and practice of nursing staff towards infection control measures in a tertiary care hospital", *Journal of the Academy of Hospital Administrations*, Vol. 13, No. 2, pp. 31–35.

Viswanathan, S. (2002a) "Do ISO certified hospitals really follow the standards?", *Express Healthcare Management*. Available at: http://www.expresshealthcaremgmt.com/20020815/cover1.shtml

Viswanathan, S. (2002b) "Karnataka takes lead with ISO for government hospitals", *Express Healthcare Management*. Available at: http://www.expresshelathcaremgmt.com/20020430.shtml

Walshe, K., L. Wallace, T. Freeman, L. Latham and P. Spurgeon (2001) "The external review of quality improvement in health care organizations: A qualitative study", *International Journal for Quality in Health Care*, Vol. 13, No. 5, pp. 367–374.

Walters, D. and S. Jones (2001) "Value and value chains in health care: A quality management perspective", *The TQM Magazine*, Vol. 13, No. 5, pp. 319–333.

Weingart, S.N., R. McL Wilson, R.W. Gibberd and B. Harrison (2000) "Epidemiology of medical error", *BMJ*, Vol. 320, pp. 774–777. Available at: http://bmj.bmjjournals.com/cgi/content/full/320/7237/774

Wensing, M. and G. Elwyn (2003) "Improving the quality of health care: Methods of incorporating patients' views in health care", *BMJ*, Education & Debate, Vol. 326, pp. 877–879.

West, E. (2001) "Management matters: The link between hospital organization and quality of patient care", *Quality in Health Care*, Vol. 10, No. 1, pp. 40–48.

WHO (1993) "The contemporary use of standards in health care", Division for Strengthening of Health Services & District Health Systems, Geneva: World Health Organization.

WHO (2000) "Health systems: Improving performance", The World Development Report 2000, Geneva: World Health Organization.

Wocher, V.J.C. (1997) "Efforts in Japanese hospitals: Why not?", in *The Effectiveness of CQI in Health Care: Stories from a Global Perspective*, V.A. Kazandjian (ed.), ASQC Health Care Series, Milwaukee, Wisconsin: ASQC Quality Press, pp. 49–108.

World Development Report (2004) The World Bank, Washington D.C.

Xie, M., K.C. Tan, S.H. Puay and T.N. Goh (1998) "A comparative study of nine National quality awards", *The TQM Magazine*, Vol. 10, No. 1, pp. 30–39.

Yang, C. (2003) "The establishment of a TQM system for the health care industry", *The TQM Magazine*, Vol. 15, No. 2, pp. 93–98.

Zabada, C., P. Asubonteng Rivers and G. Munchus (1998) "Obstacles to the application of total quality management in health-care organizations", *Total Quality Management*, Vol. 11, No. 1, pp. 57–66.

Zairi, M. and Y.F. Jarrar (2001) "Measuring organizational effectiveness in the NHS: Management style and structure best practices", *Total Quality Management*, Vol. 12, Nos. 7–8, pp. 882–889.

Zeithaml, V., A. Parashuraman and L.L. Berry (1990) *Delivering Quality Service*, New York: Collier Macmillan.

Zhang, Z., A. Waszink and J. Wijngaard (2000) "An instrument for measuring TQM implementation for Chinese manufacturing companies", *International Journal of Quality & Reliability Management*, Vol. 17, No. 7, pp. 730–755.

Zhu, Z. and L. Scheuermann (1999) "A comparison of quality programmes: Total quality management & ISO 9000", *Total Quality Management*, Vol. 10, No. 2, pp. 291–297.

Index

accreditation, 6, 34
  in healthcare organizations, 34–36, 75–80, limitations of, 36–37
  in India, 6, 34
Adinolfi, P., 9, 12, 102
Aggarwal, A.K. and M. Zairi, 4, 144
Ahire, S.L., D.Y. Golhar and M.A. Waller, 11, 114, 144, 147, 148, 194
Andaleeb, S.S., N. Siddiqui and S. Khandakar, 106, 194
Anderson, D.J., R.G. Norton, G.E. Reed and J.W. Moran, 9
Ang, C., M. Davies and P.N. Finlay, 11, 102, 114, 148, 160, 194
Arya, S.K., D.K. Sharma, S.S. Nagarajan and V. Kaushal, 13, 88
audit methods
  cycle of, 38
  for medical services, 37–38, problems of, 38–39

Bedi, S., S. Arya and R.K. Sarma, 84, 88
Beecham, L., 39
Benneyan, J.C., R.C. Lloyd and P.E. Plsek, 26
Berman, P. and P.R. Eliya, 75
Berman, Peter, 4
Bharat, R., 84
Bharat, V., 73
Bharat, V., B. Mohanty and N.K. Das, 9, 84, 88, 144
Bhardwaj, A., D.K. Sharma, R.K. Sarma and P.C. Chaubey, 13, 184
Bhat, R., 77
Black, S.A. and L.J. Porter, 11, 102, 104, 115, 118, 147, 194
Boyce, N., 20
Brown, R.B. and L. Bell, 7, 38, 39
Buchan, H., 20

Caldwell, C., 9
Carman, J.M., 27
Castle, N.G., 59
Chanda, R., 2
Chang, C. and B. Cheng, 9
Chassin, M.R. and R.W. Galvin, 5
Chow-Chua, C. and M. Goh, 9, 13, 104, 170

CII-McKinsey, 2, 3
Clarke, A., 69
clinical audit, 37
clinical governance, 39
principles of, 39–40
Coddington, D.C., L.E. Palmquist and W.V. Trollinger, 18
Collingwood, M.P., 27, 44
Collins, C.D., D.J. Hunter and A.T. Green, 37
Continuous Quality Improvement (CQI), 32
corporatization of healthcare, 54
Counte, M.A. and S. Meurer, 11, 102, 115, 118, 147, 168
Cuganeshan, S., G. Bradley and P. Booth , 12, 96
Cunha, M.P.E., J.V.D. Cunha and S. Dahab, 64

Das, N.K., S. Prasad and K. Jayaram, 88
DesHarnais, S.I. and C.P. McLaughlin, 25, 35, 36
Dhanjal, H., 88
Donaldson, L.J. and J.A.M. Gray, 37, 39

Eggli, Y. and P. Halfon, 7, 36, 42

Flynn, B.B. and B. Saladin, 11, 102, 104, 115, 118

Gaucher, E.J. and R.J. Coffey, 4, 9, 20, 23, 65, 92, 101
Ghobadian, A. and H.S. Woo, 98, 99, 168
Ginter, P.M., L.E. Swayne and W.J. Duncan, 4, 20
Goonan, K. Jennison , 23, 126, 127
Gupta, A., 83, 88, 91
Gupta, S.K. and S. Kant, 84
Gyani, G.J. and M.B. Mittal, 40

Haigh, D., 50
Harteloh, P.P.M., 25, 46
health sector reforms, 4–5
need for, 19–21
healthcare accreditation schemes
in the UK, 34
healthcare expenditure/ spending, 2
at the global level, 4
in India, 2–3, 72
in the US, 4
healthcare industry, 1, 2, 54
accreditation in, 7–8
in India, 1, growth in, 1–2, 71–75, 184; market size and trends, 3
quality management in, 5, barriers to, 92–94
healthcare quality, 25, 30, 31
barriers to maintain, 92–94
concept of, 18
core issues in defining, 21–22
need for, 18, 19–21
technical aspects of, 22–24
healthcare services, 17
in India, growth of, 71–75; regulation and accreditation of, 75–80; quality management in, 74–75
healthcare system, 1
in the US, 4
objectives of, 2
quality in, 5, improvement of, 45–48
Hewison, A., 4
Hind, M., 7, 43

Houghton, G. and D. Wall, 40
Huq, Z., 4, 9, 12, 20, 104, 115, 194
Hurst, K., 7, 34, 37

IBEF, 2
India's Service Revolution, 1, 185
Indian Medical Association, 76
industrialization of healthcare, 54
ISO certification, 7, 40
  categories of, 40–41
  for hospital, 40–43
  limitations of, 42–43

Jain, S.K. and G. Gupta, 5
Jesani, A., 77

Kandampully, J. and L. Butler, 18
Kanji, G.K. and P.M.E. SÁ, 10, 13, 115, 170
Kant, S. and S.K. Gupta, 88
Kazandjian, V.A., 9, 20
Klein, D., J. Motwani and B. Cole, 9
Köeck, C.M., 24
Krüger, V., 50
Kumar, K., R. Subramanian and C. Yauger, 18
Kunst, P. and Lemmink, J. , 10, 13, 65, 102, 104, 114, 115, 144, 186, 189, 194

Lakhe, R.R. and R.P. Mohanty, 11, 114, 172
Leatherman, S. and K. Sutherland, 37, 39
Lin, B. and J. Clousing, 12, 102, 144
Logothetis, N., 50
Low, S.P., 7, 42
Lozano, A.R.P., 42,

Macdonald, J., 24
Magd, H. and A. Curry, 7, 42
Mahapatra, P., S. Sinatra and P. Sridhar, 13, 84
Mandal, P., P.E.D. Love, A.S. Sohal and B. Bhadury, 114
Manjunath, U., 30, 180
Manjunath, U., A.K. Bhat and N.V.M. Rao, 106
Mathews, B. and M.C. Clark, 95
McLaughlin, C.P. and A.D. Kaluzny, 9, 12, 28, 50, 52, 54, 55, 57, 59, 62, 101, 115, 187
McLaughlin, C.P. and K.N. Simpson, 20, 65, 68
medical audit, 37
  drawbacks of, 38–39
  methods of, 37–38
Medical Council of India, 75
medical services, 17
Meyer, S.M. and D.A. Collier, 13, 102, 104, 113, 115, 118, 144, 159, 194
Mitra, S., 83, 88
Mohanty, R.P. and R.R. Lakhe, 50
Mohanty, R.P., K. Santi and C. Haripriya, 18, 144
Moody, D., J. Motwani and A. Kumar, 9
Motwani, J., 172
Mukherjee, A., 76

NABH, 79
Naidu, A., 105, 194
Nandaraj, S., A. Khot, S. Menon and R. Brugha, 7, 114

Nandraj, S., 77
Nandraj, S., A. Khot and S. Menon, 73
Nandraj, S., N. Madhiwala, R. Sinha and A. Jesani, 78
Narang, R., 194
National Health Policy (NHP), 2002, 2–3
National Health Service (NHS) of Great Britain, 4
National Rural Health Mission, 80
Newman, K., 37
Nunnaly, J.C., 155

organizational standards
  categories of, 33
outcome quality, 25
Øvretveit, J. and D. Gustafson, 12, 69, 102, 118
Øvretveit, J., 8

Parasuraman, A., V.A. Zeithaml and L.L. Berry, 12, 27, 93, 94, 95
Phadke, A., 73, 75
Potter, C., P. Morgan and A. Thomson, 6, 32, 43
Priebe, S., 7, 28, 42
private health services
  in India, 72, 73
process quality, 24
public health system
  in India, 80, quality initiatives in, 80–82

Quality Assurance (QA), 6, 32
  and TQM, difference between, 45–66
  in healthcare, 32–33, mechanisms for, 33–43
  limitations of, 43–45
  mechanism(s) for, 32
quality awards, 98
  aims of, 99
  role of, in TQM, 98
quality gurus, 50, 53–54
quality in fact, 27
quality in perception, 27
quality management
  in healthcare organizations, 5, approaches to, 6, 32; improvement in, 45–48
  methods of, 10; barriers to, 92–94
quality of care, 18
  in medicine field, 18, 31
quality, 5, 21, 54
  components of, 28
  concept of, 5, 30, 184
  in healthcare systems, 5–6, 21
  levels of, 28
  management of, at the organizational level, approaches to, 6, 32

Rabbani, F., S.M. Wasim Jafri, F. Abbas, F. Jahan, N. Syed, G. Pappas, S.I. Azam, M. Brommels and G. Tomson, 106, 194
Raja, M.P.N., S.G. Deshmukh and S. Wadhwa, 104, 194
Ramani, K.V. and D. Mavalankar, 4, 73
Rameshan, P. and S. Singh, 84, 88
Rao, A.T. and A.K. Agarwal, 82
Reddy, B.K. and G.V.R.K. Acharyulu, 13, 88
Reddy, B.K., M. Arundhathy and G.V.R.K. Acharyulu, 13, 82
Reichheld, F.F. and W.E. Sasser, 9
Ritchie, L., 37, 39
Ruyter, K.D. and M. Wetzels, 96

Sahni, A., 88
Samaddar, D.P., S. Kumar, A. Sunder, B. Ray, A. Ahmed, S. Sreedevi and P.K. Sahu, 84
Saraph, J.V., P.G. Benson and R.G. Schroeder, 11, 101, 104, 114, 144, 145, 147, 160, 194
service sector, 1
  in India, 1, growth of, 1
Shaw, C.D., 33, 37, 40
Short, P.J. and M.A. Rahim, 10, 21, 33, 45, 47, 92
Sila, I. and M. Ebrahimpour, 11, 12, 114, 115
Singhal, S., R. Tata, M. Kar, R. Sinha, S. Trivedi and G. Jaganath, 9, 84
Sureshchandar, G.S., C. Rajendran and R.N. Anantharaman, 12, 89, 102, 104, 114, 115, 144, 147, 148, 169, 187, 189, 194
Sutcliffe, K.M., 22
Sutherland, K. and S. Dawson, 37, 39

Tabish, S.A., 4
Tan, K.C., 114
Tarí, J.J., 7, 11, 43, 114
Thomson, R.G. and K. Hodgson, 6, 7, 20, 33, 37, 39, 58
Total Quality Management (TQM), 8, 47
  and QA, difference between, 45–46
  as a method of leadership and management, 47–48
  concepts of, 49–54
  elements of, 59, 60–61
  implementation of, critical factors for, 11–14
  in healthcare, 8–11, 49, 50, 54–58, general framework of, 59–64; advantages of, 64–69
  of hospitals, in India, 82–84
  role of quality awards in, 98–101
total quality revolution, 9
Total Quality Service (TQS), 12, 91
  in India, research gaps in, 84–89

Varghese, R., 13, 88
Verma, D.P.S. and R. Sobti, 13, 84, 88
Vij, A., S.N. Williamson and S. Gupta, 84
Viswanathan, S., 8, 81

Walshe, K., L. Wallace, T. Freeman, L. Latham and P. Spurgeon, 6, 8, 32, 33, 44, 45,
Weingart, S.N., R. McL Wilson, R.W. Gibberd and B. Harrison, 20
WHO, 7
Wocher, V.J.C., 98

Xie, M., K.C. Tan, S.H. Puay and T.N. Goh, 99

Zabada, C., P. Asubonteng Rivers and G. Munchus, 62, 92
Zairi, M. and Y.F. Jarrar, 37
Zhang, Z., A. Waszink and J. Wijngaard, 11, 104, 114, 145, 148, 160, 194
Zhu, Z. and L. Scheuermann, 7, 43